Minimum System Requirements
PC
CPU:Pentium III or higher
64 MB Ram; 128 MB Ram preferred
800 x 600 monitor with thousands of colors
OS: Windows/2000/XP
8x CD-ROM drive
135 MB hard disk space

LICENSE AGREEMENT

D0024818

LIMITED WARRANTY AND DISCLAIMER

FAD warrants that the CD-ROM on which the Software is furnished will be free from defects of sixty (60) days from the date of delivery to you by FAD or FAD's authorized representative of distributor. Your receipt shall be evidence of the date of delivery. The Software and accompanying materials are provided "as is" without warranty of any kind. The complete risk as to quality and performance of a nonwarranted program is with you.

FAD makes no warranty that the Software will meet your requirements or that Software operation will be uninterrupted or error free or that Software defects are correctable. No oral or written information or advice given by FAD, its dealers, distributors, agents, or employees shall create warranty or in any way increase the scope of this limited warranty.

REMEDIES. FAD's entire liability and your exclusive remedy shall be limited to replacing the defective media if returned to FAD (at your expense) accompanied by dated proof of purchase satisfactory to FAD not later than one week after the end of the warranty period, provided you have first received a Return Authorization by calling or writing FAD in advance. The maximum liability of FAD and its licensors shall be the purchase price of the Software. In no event shall FAD and its licensors be liable to you or any other person for any direct, indirect, incidental, consequential, special, exemplary, or punitive damages for tort, contract, strict liability, or other theory arising out of the use of, or inability to use, the Software.

ENTIRE AGREEMENT. This Agreement contains the entire understanding of the parties hereto relating to the subject matter hereof and supersedes all prior representations or agreements.

GOVERNING LAW. This Agreement and Limited Warranty are governed by the laws of the Commonwealth of Pennsylvania. All warranty matters should be addressed to F.A. Davis, Publishers, 1915 Arch Street, Philadelphia, PA. 19103.

INSTALLATION INSTRUCTIONS

Windows

Step 1. Insert CD into your CD-ROM drive.

Step 2. After a few moments, the CD-ROM menu will automatically open.

Step 3. Select the item to install

If the CD-ROM Menu does not automatically open, from the START Menu, select RUN and enter X:\SETUP.EXE (where "X" is the letter of your CD-ROM drive) and select OK

For Technical Support, e-mail: support@fadavis.com

NCLEX-RN®
Notes

Core Review & Exam Prep

Barbara A. Vitale, RN, MA

Purchase additional copies of this book at your health science bookstore or directly from F. A. Davis by shopping online at www.fadavis.com or by calling 800-323-3555 (US) or 800-665-1148 (CAN)

A Davis's Notes Book

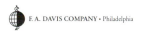

F. A. DAVIS COMPANY • Philadelphia

F. A. Davis Company
1915 Arch Street
Philadelphia, PA 19103
www.fadavis.com

Printed in China by Imago

Last digit indicates print number: 10 9 8 7 6 5 4 3 2 1

Publisher, Nursing: Robert G. Martone
Project Editor: Padraic Maroney
Manager of Art and Design: Carolyn O'Brien
Content Development Manager: Darlene Pedersen
Contributing Author: Mary Ann Hellmer-Saul, RN, AAS, BS, MS, PhD, ANP
Consultants: Paula A. Olesen, RN, MSN; Daryl Boucher, MSN, RN, CCEMTP; Golden Tradewell, PhD, RN; Kathy Whitley, RN, MSN, FNP; Leesa A. McBroom, MSN, APRN, FNP-C; Lindsey L. Carlson, MSN, RN; Eileen Kaslatas, MSN, RN; Joanne Vitale, RPA-C, BA; William Hendricks, RPh; Jean Prochilo, RN, BS; Nina Goldsztejn, RN, BC, BSN, MSN, NP

As new scientific information becomes available through basic and clinical research, recommended treatments and drug therapies undergo changes. The author(s) and publisher have done everything possible to make this book accurate, up to date, and in accord with accepted standards at the time of publication. The authors, editors, and publisher are not responsible for errors or omissions or for consequences from application of the book, and make no warranty, expressed or implied, in regard to the contents of the book. Any practice described in this book should be applied by the reader in accordance with professional standards of care used in regard to the unique circumstances that may apply in each situation. The reader is advised always to check product information (package inserts) for changes and new information regarding dose and contraindications before administering any drug. Caution is especially urged when using new or infrequently ordered drugs.

Look for our other
Davis's Notes titles

Available Now!

RNotes®: *Nurse's Clinical Pocket Guide*
ISBN: 0-8036-1335-0

LPN Notes: *Nurse's Clinical Pocket Guide*
ISBN: 0-8036-1132-3

MedNotes: *Nurse's Pharmacology Pocket Guide*
ISBN: 0-8036-1109-9

MedSurg Notes: *Nurse's Clinical Pocket Guide*
ISBN: 0-8036-1115-3

NutriNotes: *Nutrition & Diet Therapy Pocket Guide*
ISBN: 0-8036-1114-5

IV Therapy Notes: *Nurse's Clinical Pocket Guide*
ISBN: 0-8036-1288-5

PsychNotes: *Clinical Pocket Guide*
ISBN: 0-8036-1286-9

LabNotes: *Pocket Guide to Lab & Diagnostic Tests*
ISBN: 0-8036-1265-6

Contacts • Phone/E-Mail

Name:
Ph: e-mail:

Name:
Ph: e-mail:

Name:
Ph: e-mail:

Name:
Ph: e-mail:

Name:
Ph: e-mail:

Name:
Ph: e-mail:

Name:
Ph: e-mail:

Name:
Ph: e-mail:

Name:
Ph: e-mail:

Name:
Ph: e-mail:

Name:
Ph: e-mail:

Name:
Ph: e-mail:

Name:
Ph: e-mail:

NCLEX-RN®

- The National Council Licensure Examination for registered nurses (**NCLEX-RN®**) measures the knowledge and abilities necessary for entry-level nurses.
- It is administered by Computer Adaptive Testing (CAT), which individualizes tests to match the unique competencies of each test taker.
- Each exam adheres to the NCLEX-RN® Test Plan, which describes the content and scope of RN competencies.
- Practices basic to nursing (e.g., nursing process, caring, teaching, learning, communication, documentation) are integrated throughout, and most questions require application and analysis of information.

NCLEX-RN® Test Plan—Distribution of Content

Patient Needs and % of Items	
Safe and Effective Care Environment	
■ Management of Care	13%–19%
■ Safety/Infection Control	8%–14%
Health Promotion and Maintenance	6%–12%
Psychosocial Integrity	6%–12%
Physiological Integrity	
■ Basic Care/Comfort	6%–12%
■ Pharmacological/Parenteral gfd Therapies	13%–19%
■ Reduction of Risk Potential	13%–19%
■ Physiological Adaptation	11%–17%

Taking the NCLEX-RN® Test on a Computer

- First: You will receive general information about the exam and the testing center. Your time spent on this will not count.
- Second: You will take a tutorial on how to use the computer to answer the questions on NCLEX-RN®. Your answers will not count toward your score, but the time you take will be subtracted from the total 6 hours you have for the exam.
- Third: You will then be presented with real NCLEX-RN® items; there will be between 75 and 265 items. The test ends when it is 95% certain your ability is ↑ or ↓ the passing standard.

- Answers may be selected or deleted several times if desired before confirming a final answer. You must answer every question. You cannot return to a previous question.
- A time-remaining clock is in the screen's upper right-hand corner.
- A calculator on the computer is available for calculations.
- **Go to www.NCSBN.org to access an NCLEX tutorial to practice multiple choice and alternate format items on the computer.**

Critical Thinking

Definition, Influences, and Uses of Critical Thinking

- **Definition of critical thinking:** Cognitive technique by which you reflect on and analyze your thoughts, actions, decisions
- **Intellectual standards that influence critical thinking:** Focused, methodical, clear, deliberate, logical, relevant, accurate, precise
- **Processes that require critical thinking:** Test taking, nursing process, problem solving, decision making, diagnostic reasoning

Maximize Your Critical Thinking Abilities

Action	Benefit
Be positive: Be optimistic	
■ **Maintain positive mental attitude:** Replace negative thoughts with positive ones	■ ↑Positive thinking and ↓negative thinking that can interfere with learning
Be calm: Control anxious feelings	
■ **Use relaxation techniques:** Practice breathing exercises and guided imagery	■ ↓Anxiety ■ ↑Control in relation to intellectual tasks
Be inquisitive: Question and investigate	
■ **Ask the questions how, why, what:** e.g., How does Colace promote a bowel movement? Why does BP drop with hemorrhage?	■ ↑Ability to determine significance of information ■ ↑Understanding/retention of information ■ ↑Ability to apply information
Be persistent: Follow a course of action	
■ **Develop self-discipline:** Be logical and organized	■ ↑Control over variables associated with thinking

Maximize Your Critical Thinking Abilities *(Continued)*	
Action	**Benefit**
■ **Develop perseverance:** Adhere to a preset study schedule; remain determined ■ **Maintain motivation:** Set short and long-term goals; divide tasks into steps; reward self	■ ↓**Procrastination;** ↑enthusiasm ■ ↑Efficiency of time management ■ ↓Stress of making purposeful daily study decisions: inspires action ■ ↑Goal-directed behavior
Be creative: Be innovative and resourceful	
■ **Develop open-mindedness:** Compartmentalize identified beliefs, opinions, biases, stereotypes, prejudices ■ **Develop comfort with ambiguity:** Recognize that there is more than 1 way to perform a task/achieve a goal ■ **Develop independent thought:** Consider all possibilities and arrive at an autonomous conclusion ■ **Take risks:** Implement unique interventions within the definition of nursing practice and safety guidelines	■ ↑**Openness to different perspectives;** ↓egocentric thinking; ↑nonjudgmental thinking/practice ■ ↑Comprehension, synthesis, interpretation, analysis of information: promotes practice based on principles; innovation ■ ↑Ability to synthesize, summarize, conceptualize: promotes practice based on principles; ↑innovation
Be reflective: Thoughtfully explore and assess	
■ **Develop courage:** Confront difficult tasks (e.g., reviewing mistakes) with a non-judgmental attitude ■ **Develop humility:** Admit your limitations—defensive thinking promotes negativity, which closes the mind ■ **Use retrospective reviews:** Recall information/event to rediscover/explore its meaning; conduct internally or with others	■ Removes negative emotions from the task; ↑positive thinking ■ Allows an open mind to explore and acquire information; permits nonjudgmental review of mistakes ■ Identifies strengths, weaknesses, and gaps in knowledge; ↑understanding of relationships between information and its application; ↓future mistakes

General Study Skills

- Set goals
- Take class notes
- Manage your time
- Control internal and external distractions
- Establish a routine
- Simulate a school environment
- Prepare for class
- Balance sacrifices and rewards

Use Techniques Appropriate for Learning Domains

Action	Benefit

Cognitive domain (thinking): Knowing, comprehending, applying, analyzing, synthesizing, evaluating

Use all your senses	↑Reception of information
Use memorization techniques	↑Retention of basic information
Put information into your own words	↑Understanding
Apply information in new situations	Encourages correct use of information

Affective domain (feeling): Receiving, valuing, organizing, characterizing

Observe role models	↑Sensitivity
Explore feelings, beliefs, values	↑Self-disclosure/growth
Integrate values into philosophy of life	↑Consistency in actions; allows for self-actualization

Psychomotor domain (doing): Imitating, manipulating, developing precision, articulating, naturalizing

Observe others performing a skill	Identifies steps of a skill
Manipulate equipment while doing procedures	Transfers information from head to hands
Include speed/timing when practicing skills	Promotes proficiency through repetition
Practice skills repeatedly	Perfects the skill; naturalization occurs when skill becomes automatic

Specific Study Skills

How to Remember/Recall Information: Commit Facts to Memory

Action	Benefit	Example
Memorization: Repeatedly reciting out loud, reviewing in your mind, writing it down	■ Repetition ↑retention of information	■ Lists on index cards: Steps of a procedure; signs of a specific electrolyte imbalance ■ Flash cards: Drug classification on one side and action on reverse side; medical terminology on one side and definition on reverse side
Alphabet cues: Combination of significant letters	■ Each letter prompts recall of specific information	■ The 3 Ps: Cardinal signs of diabetes melitus: ■ Polyuria: Increased secretion/excretion of urine ■ Polydipsia: Excessive thirst ■ Polyphagia: Eating excessive amounts of food
Acronyms: Word formed from the first letters of a series of facts	■ Each letter jolts retrieval of specific information	■ RACE: Procedure for a fire in a health care facility ■ Rescue people in immediate danger ■ Activate the fire alarm ■ Confine the fire ■ Evacuate people to a safe area
Mnemonics: A phrase, motto, verse	■ Prompts recall of specific information	■ "There are 15 grains of sugar in 1 graham (gram) cracker." This sentence should help you remember that 15 grains are equivalent to 1 gram.

How to Understand Information: Translate, Interpret, and Determine Implications of Information

Action	Benefit	Example
Explore how or why information is relevant and valuable	■ Significant information is more likely remembered	■ Elevation of an extremity reduces peripheral edema ■ **How:** Hand held above elbow/shoulder ↑venous return via gravity, which ↓edema
Study in small groups	■ Sharing/listening ↑understanding and corrects misinformation	■ Discussing differences between hyper- and hypoglycemia ■ Debating the pros and cons of breastfeeding ■ Identify more correct things the nurse should do in addition to the correct answer presented in a test question

How to Manipulate Information: Apply, Solve, Modify, and Use Information

Action	Benefit	Example
Relate new information to prior learning	■ Placing information within a personal frame of reference makes information more meaningful	■ Pathophysiology of diabetes should build on normal physiology of the pancreas ■ Placing a pt in a left side–lying position after a liver biopsy should build on the fact that pressure compresses blood vessels, which supports hemostasis preventing hemorrhage
Recognize commonalities	■ Application of information to similar situations ↑learning	■ Actions that use the principle of gravity: Enema instillation, elevation of extremity to limit edema, high Fowler's position to promote respirations

How to Analyze Information: Examine the Organization, Structure, and Interrelationships of Information		
Action	**Benefit**	**Example**
Recognize differences	■ ↑Ability to analyze and discriminate significance of information	■ Variety of causes that can ↑BP: Hypervolemia, rigid arterial walls, emotional stress
Practice test taking	■ Reinforces learning, builds endurance, ↑test-taking and time-management skills, ↑testing comfort	■ Answer questions at the end of a chapter ■ Take a simulated test in a NCLEX prep book ■ Take a simulated NCLEX test on a computer
Review rationales for all options	■ Reinforces concepts and principles, ↑new learning, strengthens critical thinking, corrects misinformation	■ Review why the correct answer is correct ■ Review why the incorrect options are incorrect; look up additional information in textbooks
Modify test questions	■ Identify commonalities and differences, ↑opportunities for exploring content	■ Change a key word in a stem to change the focus: "Identify the pt adaptation associated with acute pain." Change the word acute to chronic and then identify if any options apply
Analyze your performance	■ Analysis identifies areas of strength, gaps in knowledge, information-processing errors, effectiveness of educated guesses, plans for future study	■ Identify number of questions answered correctly/incorrectly ■ Group questions answered incorrectly by Knowledge Deficits and Information Processing Errors (see Tab 8) ■ Identify Personal Performance Trends (see Tab 8) ■ Design a plan for future test success

Test-Taking and Study Tips

See enclosed disk for 160 examples of questions demonstrating the 15 test-taking tips and alternate format questions.

Identify positive polarity in a stem

■ Correct answer is in accord with a truth, fact, principle, or action that should be done; it attempts to determine if you can understand, apply, or differentiate correct information.

✓ Study Tip: Review content being tested; identify additional things the nurse should do.

Identify negative polarity in a stem

■ Correct answer reflects something that is false; the words **except, not, contraindicated, unacceptable, least, avoid, violate, untrue, side effect,** and **exception** indicate negative polarity. If 3 answers appear correct, you may have missed the negative word in the stem.

✓ Study Tip: Change negative word to a positive word and then answer the question.

Identify words that set a priority

■ Correct answer is what should be done *first*; the words **initial, main, primary, initially, greatest, best, first, most,** and **priority** require ranking of options from most to least desirable. If unable to identify correct answer, eliminate least desirable option and repeat again until left with a final option.

✓ Study Tip: After selecting correct answer, select what action should be done next.

Identify opposites in options

■ When 2 options reflect extremes on a continuum, frequently 1 of them is the correct answer; opposites may be obvious or obscure.

✓ Study Tip: Examples of opposites: hypo- vs. hyper-; increase vs. decrease; brady- vs. tachy-; identify what is associated with the incorrect opposite (e.g., tachycardia is associated with hyperthyroidism vs. bradycardia being associated with hypothyroidism).

Identify key words in a stem

■ Identify important word or phrase that modifies another word (e.g., early vs. late sign of shock).

✓ Study Tip: Change key words in stem; this changes focus of question and opportunities for learning.

Identify patient-centered options

■ Correct answers testing principles in the affective domain focus on feelings, choices, empowerment, and preferences.

✔ Study Tip: Examples of pt-centered options: Acknowledging: "Losing your independence must be difficult?" Offering a choice: "Would you like your bath at 7 or 10 today?" Empowering: Encourage pt to write down questions for the physician. Determining preferences: "What foods do you like to eat?"

Identify equally plausible options

■ When 2 options are similar and 1 is not better than the other, generally both are incorrect.

✔ Study Tip: Identify other equally plausible facts related to either the 3 incorrect options or the correct answer.

Identify options with "absolute" terms

■ The words *all, just, none, only, never, every,* and *always* have no exceptions; 1 of these before a statement that is true generally makes it an incorrect option. Options with absolute terms are more often incorrect.

✔ Study Tip: Examples of options to be eliminated: *Always* position an infant prone and *just* prescription drugs can cause interactions; exceptions include: *Always* maintaining an airway and focusing on the pt.

Identify the global option

■ A global option is a broad general statement, whereas the 3 other options are specific and inherently are included under the mantel of the global option.

✔ Study Tip: What else can be included under the global option?

Identify options that deny a patient's feelings, needs, concerns

■ Options that deny feelings, give false reassurance, focus on nurse, encourage cheerfulness, or change the subject cut off communication and should be eliminated.

✔ Study Tip: Examples of options to be eliminated: **Denies feelings:** "Don't cry. It is not so bad." **False reassurance:** "You'll feel better tomorrow." **Focuses on the nurse:** "The thought of dying would frighten me." Cheerfulness: "Cheer up. You are getting better."

Identify the unique option

■ When 3 options are similar in some way and 1 is different, the unique option often is the correct answer (e.g., 3 options promote a bowel movement and correct answer causes diarrhea).

✓ Study Tip: Identify additional similar or different examples of correct and incorrect options.

Identify clues in a stem

■ A word(s) in the stem that is identical, similar, paraphrased, or closely related to a word(s) in an option is called a *clang*; a clang can be obvious or obscure. Generally, an option with a clang is the correct answer.

✓ Study Tip: Identify a similar word(s) that relates to an important word in the stem (e.g., to the word *movement* in a stem consider similar words such as *activity* and *mobility* that may be found in an option).

Identify duplicate facts in options

■ If 2 or more facts are in each option and identical or similar facts are in at least 2 of the 4 options, and you can identify at least 1 fact that is correct or incorrect, you can eliminate at least 2 options.

✓ Study Tip: Identify additional facts that may be correct.

Use Maslow to identify correct option

■ Answer the question in light of Maslow's hierarchy of needs; basic physiologic needs are 1st-level needs that are a priority and are followed by needs associated with safety and security (2nd), love and belonging (3rd), self-esteem (4th), and self-actualization (5th).

✓ Study Tip: Identify an intervention associated with each level of Maslow's hierarchy of needs in relation to the question.

Use multiple test-taking tips

■ First analyze the stem for 1 or more test-taking tips. Then analyze the options for 1 or more test-taking tips. When you focus on what the stem is asking and eliminate options from consideration, you maximize the ability to select the correct answer.

✓ Study Tip: Practice answering questions at the end of a chapter or in test-taking books using the presented test-taking tips.

Alternate Format Questions and Test-Taking Tips

Alternate format questions evaluate certain knowledge more effectively than the typical multiple-choice question. They supplement multiple-choice questions, which remain the majority of questions. Any format, including the standard multiple-choice question, may include a chart, table, or graphic image. Alternate format questions are scored as either right or wrong, and partial credit is not given.

Ordered response (drag and drop) question

■ Presents a scenario or makes a statement and then lists a variety of actions or factors that must be placed in sequence or in order of priority. The sequence chosen must be identical to the correct sequence to receive credit.

✔ Test-Taking Tip: Identify the action/factor you believe should be first. Identify the action/factor you believe should be last. Evaluate the remaining 2 actions/factors and make a final determination as to which one goes second. The remaining action/factor is placed third.

Fill-in-the-blank (calculation) question

■ Requires manipulation, interpretations, or solving a problem based on presented information. It requires an intellectual skill such as computing a drug dosage, calculating an I&O, or determining the amount of IV solution to be given. The recorded answer must be identical to the correct answer to receive credit. You do not have to type in the unit of measurement.

✔ Test-Taking Tip: Before attempting to answer the question, recall information related to the question (e.g., memorized equivalents, formulas); this taps your knowledge first and limits confusion.

Multiple-response question

■ Asks a question and then lists several responses. You must identify the 1 or more responses that are correct. All correct responses must be selected to receive credit.

✔ Test-Taking Tip: Before looking at presented options, quickly review information you know about the topic. This taps your knowledge first and limits confusion after looking at presented options. Compare your list to presented options. Some of your recalled information should match. Then review the remaining presented options and determine if they are applicable. If you look at the presented options first, eliminate at least 1 or 2 you believe are wrong. Then identify at least 1 or 2 you believe are correct. Finally, evaluate the remaining options and make a determination if they are correct or not.

Hot-spot question

■ Asks a question in relation to a graphic image, picture, chart, or table. You must identify a location or analyze information on the illustration to answer the question. Your answer must mirror the correct answer exactly to receive credit.

✔ Test-Taking Tip: Read the question carefully to identify exactly what the question is asking. This limits misinterpretation and confusion. When questions reflect anatomy and physiology, close your eyes, visualize the area, briefly recall the significant structures and functions, and then look at the picture. When questions involve graphs or tables, first break them into segments for analysis and then review them as a whole.

Chart/exhibit question

■ Presents a problem and then provides a chart/exhibit that has several tabs. Each tab has to be clicked to retrieve information contained within the tab. The data must be analyzed and the significant information gleaned from the material presented to answer the question or eliminate incorrect options. These questions require the highest level of critical thinking (analysis and synthesis).

✓ Test-Taking Tip: First identify what the question is asking, then click each tab to collect data. Dissect, analyze, and compare and contrast the information collected in light of what the question is asking. Extensive information must be recalled from your body of knowledge and compared to the information in context of the situation presented in the question.

Cardiopulmonary Resuscitation (CPR)—Child and Infant

Maneuver	Child: >1year-adolescent	Infant: <1yr
Assess for response	Tap and ask, "Are you OK?"	No response to verbal or tactile stimuli
Activate 911 1 rescuer	Witnessed collapse with no response; unwitnessed event after 5 cycles of CPR	
Airway breaths	Place on hard surface; head tilt-chin lift (lift-jaw thrust with spinal trauma); look, listen, feel for air; if not breathing, give 2 breaths; cover nose and mouth of infant when rescue breathing	
Pulse check	Carotid or femoral	Brachial or femoral
Compression landmarks	Center of chest, between nipples	Center of chest below nipples
Compression method: "Hard and fast" with chest recoil	1 hand: Heel of 1 hand 2 hands: Heel of 1 hand and heel of second hand on top	1 rescuer: 2 fingers 2 rescuers: 2 thumb-enciriling hands
Compression rate and depth	Rate: Approximately 100/min Depth: Approximately 1/3 to 1/2 depth of chest	
Comp/vent ratio	1 rescuer—30:2; 2 rescuers—15:2	
Defibrillation	Sudden collapse: ASAP All others: After 5 cycles of CPR	No recommendation for infants <1yr
Rescue breathing	Pulse with no breaths: >60/min: 12 to 20 breaths/min; <60/min: continue CPR	

Ethical and Legal Foundations

Basis of Ethical Decision Making

- **Autonomy:** Support personal freedom and decision making
- **Beneficence:** Promote good
- **Fidelity:** Keep promises and commitments
- **Justice:** Treat people fairly and equally
- **Nonmaleficence:** Do no harm
- **Paternalism:** Make or allow a person to make a decision for another
- **Respect:** Acknowledge rights of others
- **Veracity:** Tell the truth

Legal Terms

- **Advance directive:** Written document that addresses treatment desires in the future if unable to make decisions
- **Living will:** Specifically identifies treatment desires
- **Health care proxy (durable power of attorney):** Assigns decision making to another
- **Do not resuscitate:** Order stating that a patient should not be revived; at request of patient when able; health care proxy, family member, or legal guardian when patient is unable to give consent
- **Assault:** Threat of unlawful touching of another
- **Battery:** Unlawful touching of another without consent (e.g., procedures performed without consent)
- **False imprisonment:** Restriction/retention of patient without consent; use restraints in compliance with policy and procedure; have patient sign release if desiring to leave facility against medical advice
- **Good Samaritan Law:** Legal protection for those who render care in an emergency without expectation of remuneration
- **Libel:** Written statement causing harm to patient

- **Malpractice:** Professional negligence; occurs when the nurse owed a duty to the patient, the nurse did not carry out that duty, and it resulted in injury to the patient
- **Negligence:** Failing to perform an act that a reasonable prudent nurse would do under similar circumstances; may be an act of omission or commission. Examples: Failure to ensure patient safety (falls); improper performance of a treatment (burns from warm soak); med errors; inappropriate use of equipment (excessive IVF via pump); and failure to monitor, report, or document patient's status
- **Organ donation:** Donor card, living will, or family consent if patient is unable to participate in decision is necessary to donate organs
- *Respondeat superior:* Latin term meaning "let the master answer"; employer is responsible for acts of employee causing harm during employment activities
- **Slander:** Oral statement resulting in damage to patient; nurse incorrectly tells others that patient has AIDS and it affects patient's business
- **Uniform Determination of Death Act:**
  - **Cardiopulmonary criteria:** Irreversible cessation of circulatory and respiratory function
  - **Whole-brain criteria:** Irreversible cessation of all functions of the entire brain and brain stem (organs may be healthy for donation even though meeting whole-brain criteria)

Disease and Treatment Mnemonics

CAUTION: EARLY SIGNS OF CANCER

Change in bowel or bladder habits
A sore throat that doesn't heal
Unusual bleeding or discharge
Thickening or lump
Indigestion; dysphagia
Obvious change in a wart or mole
Nagging cough ot hoarseness

RICE: TREATMENT FOR ACUTE INJURY

Rest; ↓stress/strain on injury
Ice; vasoconstriction ↓edema and pain
Compression; external pressure
Elevate: gravity ↓edema

INFECT: S&S OF INFECTION

Increased pulse, respirations, WBCs
Nodes are enlarged
Function is impaired
Erythema, Edema, Exudate
Complains of discomfort/pain
Temperature – local or systemic

Therapeutic Nurse-Patient Relationship

Phases of Interaction

Phase	Nurse	Patient
Preinteraction: Begins before contact with patient	Explore personal feelings, values, attitudes Collect data about patient Plan for 1st interaction	Patient has no role in this phase
Orientation (introductory): Begins at first meeting of nurse/patient	Listen; be empathetic Identify boundaries of relationship (termination begins here) Clarify expectations Establish rapport	Recognize need for help Commit to a therapeutic relationship Begin to test relationship
Working: Begins when patient identifies problems to be worked on	Assist with exploration of issues Support healthy problem solving Assist with strategy development Identify own reactions to client based on own needs, conflicts, relationships **(counter transference)**	Develop trust in nurse Examine personal issues Develop strategies to resolve issues May superimpose feelings from another relationship onto the nurse/patient relationship **(transference)**
Resolution (termination): Begins when problems are resolved; ends when relationship is terminated	Review objectives/goals achieved Reinforce adaptive behaviors Share feelings about termination Avoid discussing previous issues Encourage independence; focus on future Promote positive family interactions Refer to community resources	Share feelings about termination (anger, rejection, regression; negative feelings may be expressed to deal with loss) May attempt to discuss previous issues Assume responsibility for use of community resources

Interviewing

Interviewing Skills

- **Active listening:** Absorbs content/feelings; uses all senses; includes verbal/nonverbal attending, appropriate gestures (head nodding), eye contact, sitting, open posture, vocal cues ("mmm").
- **Clarification:** Asks for more information. Checks accuracy. ↓Ambiguity: "I am not sure I know what you mean by that."
- **Confrontation:** Presents reality, identifies inconsistencies. ↑Self-awareness. Use gently after trust is developed. Pt: "I never have any visitors." Nurse: "I was here yesterday when you had 3 visitors."
- **Direct:** Collects specific information quickly: "Where is your pain?"
- **Focusing:** Let patient finish thoughts. Centers on key elements to content; encourages discussion. Pt: "When talking about your house, you mentioned scatter rugs. Let's talk more about being safe in your home."
- **Nonverbal:** Promotes verbalization. Techniques include leaning forward, nodding head, smiling, gestures.
- **Open-ended:** Invites elaboration, nonthreatening. Avoids yes/no answer: "Tell me about what a typical day is like for you."
- **Paraphrasing:** Restates message in same/similar words. Focuses on content; encourages discussion. Pt: "I may not make it through the surgery." Nurse: "You think you are going to die?"
- **Reflection:** Describes/interprets feelings/mood: "You sound upset."
- **Silence:** Allows time for reflection, processing a response. Prompts talking. Useful when patient is sad/grieving or remaining quiet.
- **Summarizing:** Reviews key elements; brings closure. Clarifies expectations: "Today we talked about . . ."
- **Touch:** Conveys caring, is reassuring. May invade personal space; avoid with suspicious or angry patients. Hold patient's hand, patting gently on patient's shoulder.
- **Validation:** Confirms what the nurse has heard or observed: "I understand that you just said . . ."

Barriers to Communication

- Pain
- Failing to listen
- Overly optimistic statements (false reassurance)
- Advising
- Changing topic
- Judgmental or minimizing comments

- Challenging, defensive, or disapproving responses
- Direct probing and "how" and "why" questions
- Interruptions, environmental noise, or extremes in temperature
- Trite, common expressions (clichés)

Leadership

Leadership and Management Terms

- **Accountability:** Answerable for actions/judgments regarding care
- **Autonomy:** Nurse can make independent decision to decide/act
- **Case management:** Coordination of interdisciplinary care for pt
- **Decentralized management:** Staff participate in decision making
- **Performance appraisal:** Evaluation of a nurse's compliance (quality & quantity) with standards and roles within job description
- **Professional standards:** Actions consistent with minimum safe professional conduct. Description of responsibilities. ANA, JCAHO, agency policy and procedure
- **Quality improvement:** Activities to ↑achievement of ideal care
- **Responsibility:** Duties and activities that nurse is hired to perform

Leadership Styles

- **Autocratic:** Complete control over decisions, goals, plan, and evaluation of outcomes; firm, insistent; often used in emergencies or when staff is inexperienced or new
- **Democratic:** Participative; shares responsibilities; uses role to motivate staff to achieve communal goals (**shared governance**), encourages intercommunication and contributions; used to help staff grow in abilities; ↑motivation, ↑staff satisfaction
- **Laissez-faire:** Nondirective; relinquishes control & direction to staff; best used with experienced, expert, mature staff who know roles

Tasks That May Not Be Delegated to Unlicensed Nursing Personnel

- Assessing, analyzing, and interpreting data
- Identifying nursing diagnoses
- Formulating a plan of care
- Evaluating pt responses to nursing care and extent of outcome achievement
- Screening and classifying pts to determine priority to receive intervention (triage)

- Giving/monitoring parenteral medications
- Performing patient teaching
- Performing professional procedures (e.g., sterile irrigations, insertion of urinary catheter, colostomy irrigation, tracheal suctioning)

Leader and/or Manager Qualities

Effective leaders and managers need to:

- **Understand human behavior**
  Have insight into its relationship to beliefs, values, feelings; be sensitive to others' feelings and problems
- **Use effective communication skills**
  Be clear, concise; avoid ambiguity; use appropriate format (verbal, written, formal, informal); be aware of own nonverbal behavior; support staff in growth of skills
- **Use power appropriately**
  Power attained through place in table of organization (positional); power attained through knowledge and experience or perceived by staff (professional); do not abuse
- **Respond to staff needs**
  Listen attentively; attend to needs; provide positive feedback; avoid favoritism; set realistic expectations; avoid mixed messages; and treat staff with respect; Counsel privately; keep promises; avoid threats, superior attitude, criticism, or aggressive confrontation
- **Delegate appropriately**
  Right person (competent subordinate), **right task** (is within scope of practice), **right situation** (nursing assistant should not perform a routine task on an acutely ill patient), **right communication** (clear instructions, validate understanding of instructions), **right supervision** (monitor actions, evaluate outcomes, review with subordinate); leader retains accountability
- **Provide opportunities for personal growth**
  Aid less experienced nurse to 'know' knowledge, experience, responsibility (e.g., mentor/preceptor, continuing education, staff education)
- **Use critical thinking and problem solving**
  Process requires effective communication, assessment, planning, and participation of staff and evaluation of outcomes
- **Recognize conditions that are conducive to change**
  Need is recognized by all staff and all have a stake in outcome; include all creativity in the process; focus on benefits; provide positive feedback; offer incentives
  - Process follows problem-solving process

- Change is planned and introduced gradually
- Change is initiated in a calm rather than chaotic atmosphere; best after a prior successful change
- Resistance is recognized and addressed; causes of resistance: change is threatening; lack of understanding; disagreeing with purpose/approach, beliefs, and values; ↑in responsibility; habit; fear of failure

Levels of Management

- **First-level**: Supervises nonmanagerial staff; oversees day-to-day activities of a group (e.g., Team Leader, Charge Nurse)
- **Middle-level**: Supervises a group of first-level managers (e.g., Supervisor, Coordinator, Head Nurse)
- **Upper-level**: Organizational executives; sets goals and strategic planning (e.g., VP for Nursing, Associate Director of Nursing)

Staff Nurse Role

- Function as role model regarding professional conduct
- Receive report from nurse previously responsible for patient
- Make rounds on all pts immediately after receiving report
- Set priorities regarding pt needs: Immediate threat to survival (problems with breathing, VS, ↓LOC), requests for help (pain, toileting), urgent but not immediate needs (teaching)
- Coordinate and/or perform care for assigned pts; use time-management skills; complete all care assigned
- Delegate care to subordinates that is within their job description
- Monitor care delegated; establish clear expectations; encourage communication; evaluate patient outcomes related to delegated tasks (nurse retains accountability for delegated tasks)
- Give report to next nurse responsible for patient
- Engage in quality improvement (QI) activities
- Participate in intradepartmental and interdepartmental meetings

Nurse Manager Role

- Function as a role model regarding professional conduct
- Set standards of performance; establish goals for the unit with the staff; mobilize staff and agency resources to attain goals
- Support mutual trust; treat staff with respect; counsel privately
- Empower staff: Support innovation, seek staff members' opinions, promote professional environment and growth, reward growth
- Perform pt rounds with multidisciplinary team

- Monitor nursing practice and achievement of standards
- Design and implement a quality improvement (QI) program for the unit; engage staff in QI activities
- Assist in staff development plan and orientation of new employees
- Schedule staffing for the unit
- Conduct regular staff meetings with all shifts
- Evaluate performance of subordinates (performance appraisal)
- Participate in intradepartmental and interdepartmental meetings

Community Nursing

- **Community health nursing (public health nursing):** Nursing care for a specific population living in the same geographic area, or groups having similar values, interests, and needs. Aims to develop a healthy environment in which to live
- **Public health functions:** Community assessment, policy development, and facilitating access to resources. Cohesiveness is promoted by engaging community members in the problem-solving process and promoting empowerment through education, opportunities, and resources. Successful public health programs are congruent with that of the interests and goals of the community
- **Assessment of a community:**
- **Structure (milieu):** Geographical area, environment, housing, economy, water, and sanitation
- **Population:** Age and sex distribution, density, growth trends, educational level, cultures and subcultures, religious groups
- **Social systems:** Education, communication, transportation, welfare, and health care delivery systems; government and volunteer agencies
- **Community-based nursing:** Nursing care delivered in the community while focused on a specific individual's or family's health care needs. The individual is viewed within the larger systems of family, community, culture, and society
- **Vulnerable populations:** People at risk for illness (e.g., homeless, living in poverty, migrant workers, living in rural communities, pregnant adolescents, suicidal individuals, frail older adults)
- **Stigmatized groups:** People viewed with disdain/disgrace (e.g., pts with dx of HIV positive, substance abuse, mental illness)
- **Settings in which nurses work:** Homes, community health centers, clinics, industry, rehabilitation centers, schools, crisis intervention centers (phone lines), shelters, halfway houses, sheltered workshops, day care centers, forensic settings

- **Roles of nurses:** Discharge planner, case manager, counselor, and epidemiologist, health promoter, case finder, caregiver, educator, researcher, consultant, advocate, role model, change agent
- **Hospice care:** Palliative (relieve or ↓discomfort) and supportive care for dying persons and their caregivers. Experts in pain and symptom management. Focuses on preserving dignity and quality over quantity of life. Supports bereavement; usually during last 6mo of life
- **Respite care:** Temporary care for homebound so that caregivers have relief from day-to-day responsibilities

Patient Education

Learning Domains

Cognitive domain: Thinking, acquiring, comprehending, synthesizing, evaluating, storing, and recalling information.

- Build on what pt knows. Present essential information first. Add information as pt asks questions.
- Teaching strategies: Lecture, discussion, audiovisuals, printed material, computer-assisted and Web-based instruction.
- Evaluation: Assess knowledge by verbal/written means.

Affective domain: Addresses attitudes, feelings, beliefs, values. Takes time to internalize need-to-change behavior.

- Understand own value system. Respect uniqueness of each pt. Help pt explore feelings.
- Teaching strategies: Discussion, play, role modeling, panel discussion, groups, role-playing.
- Evaluation: Evidence of behavior incorporated into lifestyle.

Psychomotor domain: Addresses physical/motor skills. Requires dexterity and coordination to manipulate equipment. Ultimately performs a task with skill.

- Achieve mastery of each step before moving on to next step.
- Teaching strategies: Audiovisuals, pictures, demonstrations, models.
- Evaluation: observation of performance of skill (return demonstration).

Teaching and Learning—General Concepts

- Education can prevent illness, promote or restore health, ↓complications, ↑independence and coping, ↑individual and family growth. Incorporate throughout health care delivery.
- Environment should be conducive to learning: Private, quiet, well lit, comfortable, and lack distractions (close door/curtain, shut off TV).
- Teaching process should follow format of Nursing Process.

- Both short- and long-term goals should be set to ↑motivation and allow for evaluation. Goals must be pt centered, specific, measurable, realistic, and have a time frame.
- A variety of teaching strategies that use different senses should be used (written materials, videos, discussion, demonstration).
- Teaching can be formal/informal, individualized, or within a group
- Information should move from the simple to complex, from known to unknown; be appropriate for pt's cognitive and developmental level.
- Shorter more frequent sessions most effective (15–30min)
- Learning is ↑ with repetition, consistency, practice.
- Evaluation and documentation are essential elements of teaching.

Patient Factors That Influence Learning

Culture, religion, ethnicity, and language: Commonalities and differences exist between cultures and among people from within the same culture.
- Be culturally sensitive and nonjudgmental.
- Avoid assumptions, biases, and stereotypes. Seek help from multicultural team.
- Provide teaching in pt's language. Use professional translator.

Knowledge and experience: Can promote or deter learning.
- Identify what patient already knows. Build on this foundation.
- Explore concerns related to experiences. Correct misconceptions.

Literacy: Years in school may not accurately reflect reading ability.
- Assess ability to read and comprehend material (confusion, nervousness, excuses may indicate ↓ability to read). Use illustrations, models, videos/films, discussion.
- Provide privacy.

Developmental level:
- **Children:** The younger the child the shorter the attention span. May regress developmentally when ill. Imagination can ↑fear and misconceptions. Toddlers and preschoolers are concrete thinkers; school-age children are capable of logical thinking.
  - **Nursing:** Identify developmental age to determine appropriate strategies and tools (dolls, puppet play, role playing, drawing, games, and books). Use direct, simple approach. Also direct teaching to parents.
- **Adolescents:** Need to be similar to peers. Seeking autonomy. Focused on the present.
  - **Nursing:** Be open and honest about the illness. Respect opinions and need to be like peers. Support need for control. Learning must have immediate results.

- **Adults:** Need to be self-sufficient and in control.
  - **Nursing:** Assess for readiness. Learning most effective when self-directed, built on prior knowledge and experience, and has a perceived benefit.
- **Older adults:** Needs are highly variable. Functional changes, stress, fatigue, and chronic illness can ↓learning. Changes that may occur include slower cognition, slower reaction time, becoming overwhelmed with too much detail, and ↓ability to recall new information.
  - **Nursing:** Do not underestimate learning ability. ↓Pace of teaching to allow more time to process information and make decisions. Plan shorter, more frequent teaching sessions. Teach main points and avoid irrelevant details.

Readiness to learn: Receptiveness to learning.

- Patient has to recognize the need to learn and be physically and emotionally able to participate.
- Depression, anxiety, anger, denial will interfere with readiness, motivation, and concentration.
- Pain, acute/chronic illness, O_2 deprivation, fatigue, weakness, and sensory impairment can interfere with learning.
  - Identify readiness (pt states misconceptions, asks questions, demonstrates health-seeking behaviors, is physically comfortable, and anxiety < mild).
  - Select teaching aids appropriate for pt's sensory limitations.
  - Postpone teaching until pt is able to focus on learning; address factors that interfere with learning.

Motivation: Drive that causes action. Essential to learning.

- Personal desire to learn (intrinsic motivation, internal locus of control) such as feeling better after stopping smoking.
- Desire to learn because of an external reward (extrinsic motivation, external locus of control) such as ↑salary.
- Be sincere and nonjudgmental, ensure material is meaningful, make contractual agreement, and set short-term goals to ensure success.
- Identify/praise progress (positive reinforcement), avoid criticism (negative reinforcement), allow for mistakes.
- Use interactive strategies; do not let anxiety level climb past mild.
- Assess for ↓motivation (distraction, changing subject).

Basic Nursing Measures

Body Mechanics

- Maintain functional alignment; ↑Balance, movement, physiologic function; avoids stress on muscles, tendons, ligaments, bones, joints; avoid twisting body; use supportive devices.
- ↑Balance by keeping wt within the center of gravity; avoid reaching.
- ↑Stability by spreading feet apart to widen base of support.
- Use large muscles of legs for power; avoids back muscle strain.
- Flex knees and hold objects being lifted close to body; lowers center of gravity and keeps wt within base of support; ↑stability; ↓strain.
- Raise bed to working ht; working closely to object being lifted or moved keeps object within center of gravity.
- Use internal girdle to stabilize pelvis when lifting, pulling, stooping.
- Use body wt as a force for pushing/pulling; lean forward and backward or rock on feet; ↑strain on back.
- Pull, push, roll, slide rather than lift; face direction of movement.

Fall Prevention

- Assess for risk factors: History of falls, ↓sensory perception, weakness, ↓mobility, ↓LOC, ↑anxiety, confusion, ↓mental capacity, meds (diuretics, opioids, antihypertensives).
- Orient to bed and room; teach use of ambulatory aids and call bell; answer call bell immediately.
- Keep bed in lowest position unless receiving care.
- Raise 3 of 4 side rails; raise 4 rails if it is patient's preference or there is an order (4 raised rails are considered a restraint).
- Lock wheels on all equipment and ensure that equipment is intact.
- Keep call bell, bedside and overbed table, personal items in reach.
- Keep floor dry and free of electric cords/obstacles; use night light.
- Encourage use of grab bars, railings, rubber-soled shoes.
- Stay with patient in bathroom/shower (need MD order for shower).
- Teach fall-prevention techniques (e.g., rise slowly).
- Use monitoring device to signal attempt to ambulate unassisted.

Cardiopulmonary Resuscitation (CPR)—Adult

Assess for response	Tap and ask, "Are you OK?"
Activate 911 — 1 rescuer	Witnessed collapse with no response; unwitnessed event after 5 cycles of CPR
Airway—breaths	Put on hard surface; head tilt-chin lift (lift-jaw thrust with spinal trauma); look, listen, feel for air; if not breathing, give 2–1 second breaths
Compression landmarks	Center of chest; lower half of sternum (not over xiphoid)
Compression method	Heel of 1 hand, heel of 2nd hand on top ("hard and fast" allowing for chest recoil)
Compression rate and depth	**Rate:** Approximately 100/min; **Depth:** 1½ to 2 inches
Compression/ventilation ratio	30:2
Pulse check	Carotid
Defibrillation	**Sudden collapse:** As soon as possible **All others:** After 5 cycles of CPR
Rescue breathing	**Pulse > 60/min with no breathing:** 10 to 12 breaths/min; 1 breath every 3–5 sec **Pulse <60/min with no breathing:** Continue CPR

Fire Safety

- Stay calm; keep halls clear; do not use elevator; stay close to floor.
- Know location and use of alarms and extinguishers.
- Evacuate pts in immediate danger first and then ambulatory, those needing assistance, and finally bedbound pts.
- **Class A fire:** Wood, textiles, paper trash; water extinguisher.
- **Class B fire:** Oil, grease, paint, chemicals; dry powder and CO_2 extinguisher; water will spread fire; touching horn of CO_2 extinguisher can freeze tissue.
- **Class C fire:** Electrical wires, appliances, motors; dry powder and CO_2 extinguisher.
- **RACE: Rescue** pts in danger; **Activate** alarm; **Contain** fire (close doors/windows); **Extinguish** fire if small; Evacuate horizontally and then vertically.

Foreign Body Airway Obstruction—Child and Infant

	Child: >1year–adolescent	Infant: <1yr
Assess for extent of obstruction	**Mild:** Can cough and make sounds; **Severe:** cannot cough, make sounds, or speak; difficulty breathing; pallor; cyanosis	
Victim is conscious	**Mild:** Continue to monitor **Severe:** Abdominal thrusts until object is expelled or victim unresponsive	**Mild:** Continue to monitor **Severe:** Deliver 5 back blows and 5 chest thrusts; repeat until object is expelled or victim unresponsive
Victim becomes unresponsive	Head tilt-chin lift; inspect mouth; remove object if present in pharynx; implement CPR but always inspect for object in pharynx before attempting 2 rescue breaths and remove if present; continue CPR	

Foreign Body Airway Obstruction (FBAO)—Adult

Assess for extent of obstruction	**Mild:** Can cough and make sounds; **Severe:** cannot cough, make sounds, or speak; difficulty breathing; pallor; cyanosis. Ask, "Are you choking?" If victim nods yes, initiate abdominal thrusts
Abdominal thrusts	**Mild:** Continue to monitor; **Severe:** Abdominal thrusts until object is expelled or victim becomes unresponsive
Victim becomes unresponsive	Head tilt-chin lift; inspect mouth; remove object if present in pharynx; implement steps in CPR for adult but always inspect mouth for object in pharynx before each 2 rescue breaths

FACES Pain Rating Scale

0	1	2	3	4	5
No hurt	Hurts little bit	Hurts little more	Hurts even more	Hurts whole lot	Hurts worst

Alternate coding

0	2	4	6	8	10
0	1	2	3	4	5	6	7	8	9	10
No Pain		Mild Pain		Moderate Pain		Severe Pain		Unbearable Pain

Source: Wong-Baker FACES Pain Rating Scale. From Wong D. L., Hockenberry-Eaton, M., Willson D., Winkelstein M. L., Schwartz, P. *Wong's Essentials of Pediatric Nursing*, 6th ed. St. Louis, MO, 2001, p. 1301. Copyrighted by Mosby, Inc. Reprinted by permission.

Pain Assessment Tool

P: Provokes/point. What causes the pain? Point to the pain?

Q: Quality. Is it dull, achy, sharp, stabbing, pressuring, deep, etc.?

R: Radiation/relief. Does it radiate? What makes it better/worse?

S: Severity/S&S. Rate pain on 1–10 scale. What S&S are associated with the pain (dizziness, diaphoresis, dyspnea, abnormal VS)?

T: Time/onset. When did it start? Is it constant or intermittent? How long does it last? Sudden or gradual onset? Frequency?

Nursing Care

- **Assess pain:** Use tools/scales
- **Provide comfort:** Positioning, rest
- **Validate pt's pain:** Accept that pain exists
- **Relieve anxiety/fears:** Answer questions, provide support
- **Teach relaxation techniques:** Rhythmic breathing, guided imagery
- **Provide cutaneous stimulation:** Backrub, heat and cold therapy
- **Decrease irritating stimuli:** Bright lights, noise, ↑↓room temp
- **Use distraction (for mild pain):** Soft music; encourage TV/reading
- **Provide pharmacologic relief:** Administer meds as ordered
- **Evaluate pt response:** Document; modify plan

Restraints—Nursing Care

- Physical or chemical intervention that ↓movement
- **Purpose:** preventing falls, disrupting therapy, harming self/others
- **Physical restraints:** Devices used to ↓movement (vest, mitt, wrist, elbow, belt, mummy)
- **Chemical restraints:** Meds to calm disruptive/combative behavior that may cause harm to self/others
- **Nursing**
  - Document behavior requiring need and failure of less invasive measures to protect pt; secure daily order
  - In emergency, notify MD and get order signed within 24hr
  - Ensure functional alignment before applying
  - Follow directions (correct size, snug but does not limit respirations or occlude circulation, apply vest with V opening in front, secure tails with slipknot to bed frame)
  - Pad under wrist or mitt restraints
  - Monitor respiratory and circulatory status routinely
  - Every 1–2hr remove restraint, assess skin, and provide care, perform ROM

Visually Impaired Patient—Nursing Care

- Knock on door, greet pt by name, identify self, and explain purpose
- Do not touch until after pt understands your name and purpose
- Approach in an unhurried manner and use clear, simple sentences
- Stay within the pt's field of vision
- Orient to the room, location, and use of call bell
- Provide a predictable environment; remove all hazards
- ↑Noise and distraction in the environment; explain unusual noises
- Ensure glasses are clean, accessible, and protected when stored
- Inform of location of food on meal tray; use numbers on a clock
- Ambulate pt by walking slightly in front while pt holds your arm. Never try to push or guide from behind. Inform of doors, steps
- Make it clear to pt when the conversation is over or when leaving

Hearing-Impaired Patient—Nursing Care

- Greet pt by name, identify yourself and your purpose, ensure quiet
- Use touch appropriately to alert pt that you are about to talk
- Face pt directly; avoid turning away from pt while you are speaking; to facilitate lip reading, do not cover mouth with your hand
- Talk in a normal tone at a moderate rate; speak clearly; articulate consonants carefully; do not overly articulate; do not yell
- Use gestures and facial expression to convey message
- Encourage use of hearing aid; facilitate repair of nonworking aids
- Remove hearing aid when showering or washing the hair
- Follow manufacturer's directions to insert, remove, clean, and store aid

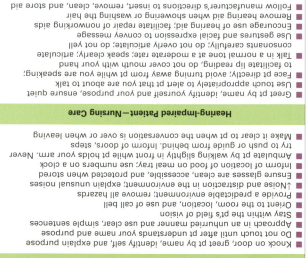

Latex Allergy

Type of Reaction	S&S	Nursing Actions
Local skin reaction: Direct skin-to-latex contact	Not life-threatening Erythema, pruritus, Popular, vesicular, scaling, or bleeding lesions;	Allergy wristband Label chart Use latex-free equipment (gloves, tape, dressings, stockings, tubing, tourniquets, stetho-scopes, electrode pads, syringes, antiembolism BP cuffs, any indwelling urinary catheters)
Excessive exposure skin-to-latex contact can lead to systemic reaction	Life-threatening Angioedema Rhinitis or rhinorrhea, Conjunctivitis Bronchospasm	
Systemic: Direct skin-to-latex contact Contact with equipment exposed to latex		

Latex Allergy *(Continued)*

Type of Reaction	S&S	Nursing Actions
Powder particles exposed to latex may be inhaled or absorbed via skin, mucous membranes, or blood	Anaphylactic responses Circulatory collapse	Notify pharmacy so meds and mixed solutions are latex-free Ensure procedure rooms are latex-free and patient is first case of day

Neutropenic Precautions

- For individuals with compromised immune system
- Use standard precautions, especially hand hygiene
- Caregivers and visitors should be free of communicable illnesses
- Private room if possible; keep room meticulously clean
- Teach to avoid sources of potential infection (crowds, confined spaces such as airplanes, raw fruits/vegetables, flowers/plants)

Sterile Asepsis

- Check expiration date; ensure packages are dry, intact, and stain-free
- Discard opened sterile solutions older than 24hr; criteria for medicated/antiseptic solutions may differ
- Place cap on table with inner cap turned up; label with date, time, and initials; avoid touching bottle rim
- Place sterile equipment inside the outer 1 inch of sterile field
- Ensure that sterile objects touch only another sterile object
- Open sterile packages away from sterile field
- Keep sterile field in one's line of vision
- Position solution closest to patient; keep field dry and free of moisture
- Don sterile gloves without contaminating sterile surfaces
- Keep sterile gloved hands and equipment above level of waist
- Avoid talking, coughing, sneezing around a sterile field
- Discard sterile objects that become contaminated or if doubtful

Standard Precautions: Tier 1

- Perform hand hygiene before and after care and when soiled; most important way to prevent infection
- Use personal protective equipment (PPE) if touching, spilling, or splashing of blood or body fluids is likely; use gloves, gowns, mask, goggles, shields, aprons, head and foot protection
- Discard disposable items in fluid-impermeable bag and contaminated items in Biohazard Red Bag
- Do not recap used needles; dispose in sharps container
- Hold linen away from body; place in impermeable bag in a covered hamper; do not let hampers overflow
- Place lab specimens in a leak-proof transport bag without contaminating the outside; label with biohazard sticker and patient information
- Institute procedure for accidental exposure: Wash area, report to supervisor, receive emergency care, seek referral for follow-up
  - Receive hepatitis B vaccine
- Assign patient to private room if hygiene practices are unacceptable
- Avoid eating, drinking, touching eyes, applying makeup in patient areas

Transition-Based Precautions: Tier 2

AIRBORNE

- Used for microorganisms that spread through air (droplet nuclei <$5\mu m$ [e.g., TB, measles, chicken pox])
- Private room; negative air pressure room; door closed; high-efficiency disposable mask (replace when moist) or particulate respirator (e.g., for TB); transport patient with mask, teach to dispose soiled tissues in fluid-impervious bag at bedside

DROPLET

- Used for microorganisms spread by large-particle droplets (droplet nuclei >$5\mu m$, (e.g., pneumonia [streptococcal, mycoplasmal, meningococcal], rubella, mumps, influenza, adenovirus])
- Private room if available or cohort pts, mask when within 3ft of pt, door open, mask for pt when transporting, teach to dispose soiled tissues in impervious bag at bedside

CONTACT

- Used for organisms spread by direct or indirect contact; methicillin-resistant S. aureus (MRSA), vancomycin-resistant enterococcus (VRE), vancomycin intermediate-resistant S. aureus (VISA); enteric pathogens (e.g., E. coli, C. difficile), herpes simplex, pediculosis, hepatitis A and E, varicella zoster, respiratory syncytial virus
- Private room or cohort pts; gowns, gloves over-gown cuffs; dedicate equipment

Nursing Care of Older Adults (>65yr)

Background

DEMOGRAPHIC DATA
- ■ 70% rate themselves as healthy. Majority live in the community; increasingly more live in assisted living facilities. 5% in nursing homes.

PHYSICAL CHANGES
- ■ Gradual ↓in physical abilities. Close vision impairment (presbyopia). ↓Hearing especially for high-pitched sounds. ↓Subcutaneous tissue. ↓Muscle strength. Impaired balance and coordination. ↓Immune response. One or more chronic health problems.

PSYCHOSOCIAL ISSUES
- ■ Conflict is ego integrity vs. despair. Personality does not change but may become exaggerated. Adjusting to aging, ↓health, maintenance of quality of life, retirement, fixed income, death of spouse/friends, change in residence, own mortality. Reminiscing may become focused on bodily needs and comforts. Sexual expression (love, touching, sharing, intercourse) important and related to identity.

COGNITIVE STATUS
- ■ IQ does not ↓. Mental acuity slows (↑time to learn, problem solve). Long-term memory better than short-term memory.

REACTION TO ILLNESS/HOSPITALIZATION
- ■ Illness/recuperation longer. Secondary to ↓adaptive capacity. ↑Feelings of inadequacy and mortality. May ↑self-absorption, social isolation, frustration, anger, depression, especially if retirement goals are denied. Unfamiliar environment may cause confusion, anxiety. Chronic illness, pain, or impending death may cause dependence, hopelessness. May accept and prepare for death.
- ■ **Nursing:** Understand commonalities of aging but approach each person as unique. Avoid stereotyping because it denies uniqueness, ↓access to care, and impacts negatively on individual. Ensure access to health care and social services, especially in home. Critical illnesses deserve aggressive treatment if desired.

Common Problems Associated With Aging

BOWEL AND BLADDER INCONTINENCE

- Not part of aging process. May be aggravated by ↓muscle tone of anal and urinary sphincters and prostatic hypertrophy.
- **Nursing:** Ensure screening for UTI, bladder/prostate cancer. Assist with hygiene and skin care. Institute bowel or bladder retraining.

ADVERSE DRUG EFFECTS

- Multiple health problems require ↑prescriptions (polypharmacy) with ↑coordination among MDs. ↑Hepatic/renal function that results in accumulation, ↑paradoxic effects.
- **Nursing:** ↑Coordination of health care. Identify unnecessary or excessive doses of meds. Assess for adverse/toxic effects.

FALLS/ACCIDENTS

- Secondary to sensory impairments (vision, hearing, touch), postural changes, ↑muscle strength and endurance, orthostatic hypotension, neurologic and cardiovascular decline.
- **Nursing:** Assist with ambulation. Teach safety precautions (use grab bars, railings, and walker; keep feet apart for a wide base; give up driving when impairment jeopardizes safety).

INFECTIONS

- Increased secondary to ↓immune response.
- **Nursing:** Teach preventive measures (handwashing, avoiding crowds, smoking cessation. Pneumococcal pneumonia vaccine, yearly flu vaccine.

COGNITIVE IMPAIRMENT

- Not part of aging process. **Delirium** is potentially reversible and is associated with acute illness. **Dementia** is a chronic, progressive, irreversible disorder. **Sundowning syndrome** is confusion after dark.
- **Nursing:** See TAB 5—Mental Health Nursing for nursing care.

ALCOHOL ABUSE

- Secondary to depression, loneliness, lack of social support.
- **Nursing:** Explore effective coping strategies. Refer to AA.

RISK OF SUICIDE

- Secondary to multiple losses (loved ones, health), lack of social support; 20% experience depression, feelings of hopelessness, and isolation.

- **Nursing:** Assess for suicide risk. Provide reality orientation, validation therapy, reminiscence. Support body image. Encourage psychological counseling; obtain order for antidepressant; referral to social service agency.

SEXUAL RESPONSIVENESS/ERECTILE DYSFUNCTION

- Sexual response takes longer; ↓estrogen and testosterone; chronic health problems; medications; unavailable partner; cognitive impairment.
- **Nursing:** Provide privacy/dignity and nonjudgmental attitude, ↑verbalization of concerns, suggest lubricants, penile prostheses, meds to reduce erectile dysfunction.

SEXUALLY TRANSMITTED INFECTIONS (STI)

- Need for sexual expression continues. ↑Society recognition that sex is natural and acceptable even if single by choice or death of spouse.
- **Nursing:** Maintain nonjudgmental attitude; teach about STI prevention.

LEADING CAUSES OF DEATH

- Heart disease, then cancer, stroke, lung disease, falls, diabetes, kidney and liver disease. Often have 1 or more chronic illnesses.
- **Nursing:** Focus on health promotion. Encourage smoking cessation, ↑exercise, wt control, adequate nutrition. Provide screening programs to identify problems early and manage chronic conditions.

Common Human Responses

Vital Signs

TEMPERATURE

- **Afebrile:** Oral: 97.5–99.5°F and rectal: 0.5–1.0°F↑ than oral route
- **Hyperthermia:** >99.5°F; **hypothermia:** <97.5°F

PULSE

- **Normal:** 60–100bpm
- **Tachycardia:** >100bpm; **bradycardia:** <60bpm
- **Thready:** Weak, feeble; **bounding:** forceful, full
- **Dysrhythmia:** Irregular pattern
- **Pulse deficit:** Difference between radial and apical rate

RESPIRATIONS

- **Eupnea, normal:** 12–20bpm
- **Tachypnea:** >20bpm; **bradypnea:** <12bpm
- **Apnea:** Absence of breathing

- **Hyperventilation:** ↑Rate and depth
- **Kussmaul:** Deep and rapid, associated with metabolic acidosis
- **Cheyne-Stokes:** Rhythmic waxing and waning from very deep to very shallow and temporary apnea
- **Orthopnea:** Upright position to breathe
- **Dyspnea:** Difficulty breathing

BLOOD PRESSURE

- **Normal:** SBP <120 and DBP < 80
- **Prehypertension:** SBP 120-139 or DBP 80-89
- **Stage 1 hypertension:** SBP 140-159 or DBP 90-99
- **Stage 2 hypertension:** SBP ≥160 or DBP ≥100

Fever

↑Temperature; low-grade fever 98.6°F–101°F; high-grade fever >101° F

S&S: Fatigue, weakness, flushed, dry skin

ETIOLOGY: Bacterial, viral, or fungal infection, DVT, med side effects, tumor

NURSING

- Monitor VS and WBC; evaluate meds for possible drug-induced fever
- Obtain diagnostic tests (sputum, blood, or urine for C&S, chest x-ray)
- Perform focused assessments: ↑Breath sounds, crackles, rhonchi, stiff neck, headache, photophobia, irritability, confusion; IV site, incisions and wounds for infection; legs for DVT (redness, warmth, swelling tenderness); urine for infection (burning on urination, cloudy, greenish/reddish color); GI S&S (diarrhea, N&V, abdominal discomfort)
- Encourage coughing and deep breathing; ↑fluid intake
- Antipyretics, tepid bath, hypothermia blanket
- Change IV site if indicated

Constipation

≤2 stools a wk and/or hard dry feces (obstruction).

S&S: Distended abdomen, rectal pressure, back pain, straining at stool, anorexia, blood-streaked stools, ↓bowel sounds

ETIOLOGY: Urge is ignored; ↓fiber in diet; ↓mobility; ↓fluids; weak abdominal or pelvic floor muscles; med side effects (opioids, iron, MAO inhibitors); anal lesions; pregnancy; laxative or enema abuse; F&E imbalance; obstruction; child: stool-withholding behavior

NURSING

- Assess stools for frequency, amount, color, consistency
- ↑Fluid intake, ↑exercise and ↑fiber in diet, binding foods (rice, bananas)
- Respond to urge; encourage sitting position and regular time each day
- ↑Relaxation and privacy; give laxatives, cathartics, enemas as ordered

Diarrhea

Passage of fluid or unformed stool >3 a day

S&S: Frequent loose stool; abdominal pain, cramps, flatus, N and V, fatigue, ↑bowel sounds, abdominal distention, anorexia; results in dehydration
ETIOLOGY: Viral, bacterial, or parasitic gastroenteritis; contaminated food or water; spicy, greasy food; raw seafood; excessive roughage; lactose intolerance; AIDS; drug side effect; anxiety; inflammatory bowel disease (ulcerative colitis, Crohn's disease); ingestion of heavy metals (lead, mercury); malabsorption syndrome

NURSING

- Assess stools for frequency, amount, color, consistency
- Assess S&S of dehydration; ↑PO fluid intake
- Assess perianal skin breakdown and provide skin care
- Assess antibiotic, stool softeners, and opiate use
- Ask about recent foreign travel and dietary intake
- Obtain stool specimen (C&S, ova, and parasite)
- Administer antibiotics, antidiarrheals, IV F & E as ordered
- Contact precautions as indicated

Hemorrhage

Bleeding that compromises tissue/organ perfusion

S&S: ↑Pulse, ↑respirations, ↓BP, narrowing pulse pressure; excessive blood loss; capillary refill >3sec; ↓peripheral pulses; cool, moist, pale, mottled, or cyanotic skin; thirst. *Early CNS S&S:* ↓LOC, anxiety, irritability, restlessness. *Late CNS S&S:* Confusion, lethargy, combativeness, coma
ETIOLOGY: *External:* Surgical and traumatic wounds. *Internal:* blunt trauma, cancer, ruptured aneurysm, GI perforation, thrombolytic therapy

NURSING

- Apply direct pressure; reinforce dressing (removal may dislodge clot)
- Monitor VS, I&O; lab results
- Maintain airway; give O₂
- Ensure #18 gauge IV access; Give IVF, blood or colloidal products

Shock

Acute circulatory collapse; ↓O_2 to cells, tissues, and organs

- **S&S:** ↓BP; ↓urinary output; capillary refill >3sec; cool, pale, mottled, or cyanotic skin; change in mental status. **Hypovolemic:** ↓Peripheral pulses. **Neurogenic:** Tachycardia or bradycardia. **Anaphylactic:** Anxiety, throat tightness, stridor, tachypnea, diaphoresis, flushing, urticaria, coma. **Septic:** Fever, tachycardia, tachypnea
- **ETIOLOGY: Hypovolemic:** Blood loss, dehydration; **Neurogenic:** Spinal cord injury, anesthesia; **Anaphylactic:** Exposure to antigen; **Septic:** Infection, endo/exotoxin release

NURSING

- **Emergency intervention:** Establish airway; suction if needed; O_2 via nonrebreather mask 10–15 L/min; supine position with legs elevated unless airway compromised, then low Fowler's; ensure IV access with 18-gauge needle; prepare for code (ex: defib), intubation, central venous access, IVF, emergency meds; transfer to ICU
- **Ongoing assessments:** ECG, hemodynamic monitoring, LOC, orientation, VS, pulse oximetry (may be unreliable due to ↓peripheral perfusion), I&O, and skin for color, temp, turgor, moistness
- **Specific to types — hypovolemic:** Control bleeding if present, volume replacement with crystalloids, colloids, plasma expanders, and/or blood products; **cardiogenic:** vasopressors, cardiotonics, antidysrhythmics; **anaphylactic:** epinephrine, antihistamines, steroids; **septic:** volume replacement, antibiotics, vasopressors, antipyretics; **neurogenic:** ensure spinal stabilization, vasopressors

Infection

Entry and multiplication of a pathogen in tissue. Can be local or systemic or can progress from local to systemic. Example: UTIs can spread to kidneys and blood stream (urosepsis). Infection is accompanied by the inflammatory response

- **S&S: Local:** Erythema, edema, tenderness, heat, ↓function; purulent exudate; positive culture. S&S also depend on tissue involved.
  Systemic: ↑VS (T, P, R, BP); chills; diaphoresis; malaise; ↑WBCs; positive culture; occasionally headache, muscle/joint pain, changes in mental status
- **ETIOLOGY:** Invasion of bacterial, viral, or fungal pathogen

NURSING

- Assess VS, S&S of inflammation and infection
- Obtain C&S before 1st dose of antibiotic if infection is suspected

- Avoid excess bed covers, change linen if diaphoretic
- Promote rest and immobilization
- Give O$_2$, IVF, ↑po fluids, ↑protein, Vit C, and wound care as ordered
- Transmission based precautions as indicated

Inflammatory Response

Local defensive vascular response to injury, infection, or allergen to protect and repair tissue; inflammatory response occurs with an infection

SIGNS AND SYMPTOMS: Histamine, prostaglandin, bradykinin, and serotonin ↑vascular permeability, causing fluids, protein, and cells to move into interstitial tissue. This causes local edema, heat, redness. Histamine irritates and edema places pressure on nerve endings → pain. Edema and pain contribute ↓function. Exudate may be clear, plasmalike (**serous**), pink with RBCs, (**sanguineous**), or yellowish-green with WBCs and bacteria (**purulent**). Purulent exudate indicates infection

ETIOLOGY: Local trauma, local infection

NURSING

- Assess for S&S of inflammation and wound characteristics
- Provide wound care as ordered
- Elevate area if possible to ↓edema. Immobilize area to ↓pain
- Give antipyretics, anti-inflammatories, antibiotics as ordered
- Apply ice (at time of injury to ↑vasoconstriction, which ↓pain/edema) or heat (after 24–48hr to ↑circulation and remove debris and localize inflammatory agents) if ordered

Nausea and Vomiting

Unpleasant wavelike sensation in throat and epigastrium (nausea). Ejection of GI contents through mouth (vomiting, emesis), which carries a risk of aspiration → atelectasis, pneumonia, asphyxiation

S&S: Nausea, vomiting, ↑↑pulse, pallor, diaphoresis, bowel sounds↑ or high pitched, abdominal pain, S&S of F&E imbalance (e.g., hypokalemia, metabolic alkalosis)

ETIOLOGY: Gastroenteritis, motion sickness, infection, pain, stress, med side effect, pregnancy, appendicitis, bowel obstruction, neurological causes (head trauma, vascular headache), ↑ICP

NURSING

- Maintain airway
- ↑HOB or place in side-lying position; keep NPO
- Assess emesis characteristics and note if vomiting is projectile

- Assess hydration status, I&O, electrolytes, daily weight
- Assess abdomen for distention and tenderness
- Attempt to determine cause
- Notify MD and obtain orders for alternate route for meds

Orthostatic Hypotension

↓BP when rising from lying down to sitting or sitting to standing secondary to peripheral vasodilation without a compensatory ↑cardiac output. Also called *postural hypotension*

S&S: Lightheadedness, vertigo, weakness; cool, pale, diaphoretic skin
ETIOLOGY: Older age, immobility, hypovolemia, anemia, dysrhythmias, med side effect (opioids, antihypertensives, diuretics)

NURSING

- Assess for ↑pulse and ↓BP when changing position
- Rise slowly, "dangle" before standing, resume prior position if dizzy
- Assist to bed, chair, or floor if falling; if ↓BP continues—assess for LOC, neurologic status, cardiac status, S&S of dehydration

Prenatal Period: Fertilization to Start of Labor

Signs of Pregnancy

- **Presumptive signs:** Absence of menses (amenorrhea); 1st awareness of fetal movement (quickening) by 16–20wk
- **Probable signs:** Softening of cervix (Goodell's sign); bluish-purple mucous membranes of cervix, vagina, and vulva (Chadwick's sign); softening of lower-uterine segment (Hegar's sign); floating fetus rebounds against examiner's fingers (ballottement)
- **Positive signs:** Fetal heart sounds; fetal movement; ultrasound of fetus

Prenatal Physiological Progression

- Ovum expelled from graafian follicle (**ovulation**); then sperm unites with ovum (**fertilization**) in fallopian tube within 24hr
- Fertilized ovum attaches to uterine endometrium (**implantation**)
- Conceptus called *embryo* (first 8wk), then *fetus*
- Trimesters: 1st (0–15wk); 2nd (16–27wk); 3rd (28–37/40wk)
- **Nägele's Rule:** Expected date of birth (EDB); add 7 days to 1st day of last menstruation, subtract 3mo, add 1yr
- Cells differentiate wk 3–8 (organogenesis); negative influences (drugs, illness) may cause defects in embryo (teratogens)
- Fetal heart audible with Doptone after 12wk
- Fetal lungs produce pulmonary surfactants at 24–28wk
- Deposits of brown fat begin at 28wk; most ↑wt in 3rd trimester
- S&S of impending labor:
  - Fetal presenting part descends into true pelvis (**lightening**)
  - Cervix thins/shortens (**effacement**); external os opens (**dilation**)
  - Mild, irregular uterine contractions (preparatory contractions, formerly Braxton Hicks)
  - Energy spurt (nesting), usually 24–48hr before labor
  - Expulsion of mucous plug, usually 24–48hr before labor

Prenatal Maternal Changes

ENDOCRINE CHANGES
- Placenta secretes human chorionic gonadotropin (hCG); used for pregnancy screening; has role in AM nausea
- Progesterone and estrogen from corpus luteum in 1st trimester; from placenta in 2nd and 3rd trimesters
- Thyroid, parathyroids, and pancreas ↑secretions; need for ↑insulin
- Estro levels ↑; excess in maternal saliva may indicate preterm labor

- Labor initiated by posterior pituitary oxytocin,↑progesterone, ↑estrogen, ↑prostaglandins

Nursing: Obtain specimens for screening tests

CIRCULATORY CHANGES
- Cardiac output ↑30–50%; blood volume ↑50%, and RBCs ↑30%
- (**physiological anemia**): ↓Hct; WBCs ↑ to 12,000mm³
- Palpitations in 1st trimester are secondary to SNS stimulation and in 3rd trimester are secondary to ↑Thoracic pressure
- HR ↑10–15 beats/min and BP drops in latter half of pregnancy; HR may ↓40% with multiple fetuses
- Supine hypotension syndrome (**vena cava syndrome**): weight of uterus on vena cava ↓venous return to heart and ↓placental blood flow; signs and symptoms include ↓BP, lightheadedness, and palpitations
- Fibrinogen and other clotting factors ↑
- Varicose veins of legs, vulva, perianal area (**hemorrhoids**) due to pressure of uterus on pelvic blood vessels
- Edema of extremities last 6wk secondary to circulatory stasis
- **Nursing:**
  - Teach patient to ↑fluids, change positions slowly, elevate legs, wear antiembolism stockings, and avoid prolonged sitting.
  - For thrombophlebitis: maintain bedrest, anticoagulant as ordered

RESPIRATORY CHANGES
- O_2 consumption ↑15% by 16–40wk
- Nasal congestion and epistaxis 2°↑estrogen levels
- Dyspnea 2° enlarged uterus pressing against diaphragm; subsides when lightening occurs around 38wk
- **Nursing:**
  - Teach to balance rest/activity; avoid large meals
  - Suggest to blow nose gently and use saline nasal spray

REPRODUCTIVE CHANGES
- Amenorrhea; leukorrhea
- ↑Vaginal acidity protects against bacterial invasion
- Cervical/uterine changes: Goodell's, Chadwick's, and Hegar's signs
- Uterus in pelvic cavity at 12–14wk and then in abdominal cavity; to umbilicus at 22–24wk and almost xiphoid process at term
- Breast changes: Fullness, tingling, soreness, darkening of areolae and nipples, nipples more erect, veins more prominent, reddish stretch marks; Montgomery's follicles enlarge
- **Nursing:**
  - Assess fundal height
  - Suggest side-lying, vaginal rear entry for intercourse
  - Tell patient not to douche and to use a supportive brassiere and cotton underpants

GASTROINTESTINAL

- Nausea without vomiting (**morning sickness**) and ↑salivation secondary to hormonal changes
- Food cravings; eating substances not normally edible (**pica**)
- Heartburn and gastric reflux secondary to delayed emptying of stomach and pressure of uterus
- Flatulence secondary to ↓GI motility, air swallowing
- Constipation secondary to ↓peristalsis, pressure of uterus, hemorrhoids
- **Nursing:**
  - Teach to avoid gastric irritants, gas-forming foods, and antacids containing Na
  - Remain upright 1hr after meals
  - Small, frequent meals; dry crackers before arising
  - ↑Fiber, fluid, and walking
  - For hemorrhoids: Avoid straining at stool and prolonged sitting, warm sitz baths or ice packs, anesthetic ointments

URINARY

- Urinary frequency in early and late pregnancy secondary to enlarging uterus
- Bladder capacity ↑ to 1500mL secondary to ↓bladder tone; may lead to stasis and infection
- ↓Renal threshold may cause glycosuria and mild proteinuria
- **Nursing:**
  - Teach to void q2h and on urge to prevent stasis
  - Assess for glycosuria secondary to DM and proteinuria $2°$ preeclampsia

INTEGUMENTARY

- Blotchy, brownish skin over cheeks, nose, and forehead (**melasma, chloasma**); pigmented line from symphysis pubis to top of fundus in midline (**linea nigra**)
- Stretch marks over abdomen, thighs, breasts (striae gravidarum) secondary to adrenocorticosteroids during 2nd half of pregnancy
- ↑Perspiration, oily skin, hirsutism, and acne vulgaris
- **Nursing:**
  - Teach that changes are common and generally subside after birth
  - Striae slowly lighten

MUSCULOSKELETAL

- Softening of all ligaments and joints, particularly symphysis pubis and sacroiliac joints; backache $2°$ lordosis, and changes in center of gravity; leg cramps $2°$ hypocalcemia and pressure of uterus on pelvic nerves
- **Nursing:**
  - Encourage intake of ↑calcium foods and perinatal vitamin
  - Teach body mechanics, avoid high-heeled shoes and lifting

NUTRITIONAL NEEDS
- 25–35lb gain: 2–5lb 1st trimester; ³/₄lb per wk 2nd–3rd trimesters
- Calories: ↑300cal/day to total of 2500cal/day
- Protein: 60 grams/day, an increase of 14 grams/day above prepregnant level
- CHO: Adequate to meet requirements; complex CHO preferred
- Fats: 30% of daily caloric intake; 10% should be saturated
- RDA vitamins and minerals attained in balanced diet and perinatal vitamin containing 400mcg folic acid; sodium is never completely restricted, avoid excess

Nursing:
- Teach patient to have a well-balanced diet, avoid dieting
- Teach patient to take a multivitamin with 400mcg folic acid daily before conception and during pregnancy to prevent neural tube defects

Prenatal Health Promotion
- **Travel:** Lap belt under abdomen and shoulder belt between breasts; stand/walk briefly q1h; airlines may restrict travel close to EDB
- **Smoking:** Avoid to prevent spontaneous abortion, ↓birth wt, apnea in newborn
- **Employment:** Avoid excessive standing or work that causes severe physical strain/fatigue
- **Alcohol:** Avoid to prevent preterm birth, ↓birth wt, fetal alcohol effects (FAE), or fetal alcohol syndrome (FAS)
- **Illicit drugs:** Avoid to prevent teratogenic effect, ↓birth wt, small for gestational age (SGA), fetal addiction, and dependency
- **Caffeine:** ↑Risk of spontaneous abortion and intrauterine growth restriction; FDA recommends ≤ 2–3 servings (200–300mg) daily
- **Artificial sweeteners:** Studies are inconclusive but moderation is recommended; mothers with PKU should avoid aspartame

Tests Performed During Pregnancy

HUMAN CHORIONIC GONADOTROPIN (HCG)
- Tests for pregnancy
- hCG is produced by cells covering the chorionic villi of placenta
- Detectable 8 days after conception
- **↑or slowly elevating levels:** Threatened abortion, ectopic pregnancy
- **↑Levels:** May indicate ectopic pregnancy, hydatidiform mole, Down syndrome

MATERNAL SERUM ALPHA-FETOPROTEIN (MS-AFP) SCREENING
- Fetal protein used to screen for neural tube defects
- Ranges identified for each wk of gestation
- Peak concentrations at end of 1st trimester
- 16–18wk optimum time for testing
- ↑Levels: Risk of open neural tube defect
- ↓Levels: Risk of Down syndrome
- When ↓levels persist, ultrasonography for structural anomalies and amniocentesis for chromosomal analysis are done

CHORIONIC VILLUS SAMPLING
- Reflects fetal chromosomes, DNA, and enzymology
- Placental tissue aspirated at 10–12wk
- Earlier testing time than amniocentesis permits earlier decision regarding termination
- Also ↓risk of 1st trimester spontaneous abortion and costs less than amniocentesis
- **Complications:** Infection, preterm labor
- **Nursing:** Obtain consent. Full bladder to serve as acoustic window. Assess VS and absence of uterine cramping. Provide emotional support. Teach spotting for 3 days is expected after transcervical route. Report flulike symptoms and vaginal discharge of blood, clots, tissue, or amniotic fluid; avoid sexual activity, lifting, or strenuous activity until spotting resolves. Ensure genetic counseling if appropriate

BIOPHYSICAL PROFILE
- Level II ultrasonography assesses FHR reactivity, fetal breathing movements and tone, amniotic fluid volume, gross body movement
- Fetus status reflected numerically like Apgar score
- Reflects CNS integrity; indicator of fetal crisis and demise
- Done in response to nonreassuring NST and signs and symptoms of fetal compromise
- **Nursing:** Same as ultrasonography; emotional support

PERCUTANEOUS UMBILICAL BLOOD SAMPLINGS (PUBS)
- Fetal cord blood assessed at >17wk. Identifies some maternal/fetal problems
- **Complications:** Bleeding, infection, thrombosis, preterm labor
- **Nursing:** Obtain consent; full bladder may be necessary; assess uterine activity, FHR, and reactivity; teach to take antibiotics and temp 2 times daily and report ↑temp

FETAL ULTRASONOGRAPHY
- Serial exams document progress, gestational age, placenta location, fetal position, and presentation

■ Assesses FHR and breathing movements, amniotic fluid index (AFI), and estimated birth wt
■ Visualizes multiple fetuses, maternal pelvic masses, gross fetal structural abnormalities, fetal demise
■ **Nursing:** Education based on findings. Provide emotional support
■ **Transabdominal:** Drink 1–2l fluid 1hr before test to fill bladder
■ **Transvaginal:** Empty bladder to ↓view of pelvic cavity

AMNIOCENTESIS

■ Analysis of amniotic fluid
■ **14–17wk:** Identifies chromosomal and biochemical disorders (e.g., Down syndrome, neural tube defects), fetal age, and gender. ↑Bilirubin signifies Rh disease, intra-amniotic infections
■ **≥35wk:** Lecithin/sphingomyelin (L/S) ratio of 2:1; phosphatidyl glycerol (PG) is present and lamellar bodies of over 35,000 particles/μL indicate lung maturity
■ **Complications:** Preterm labor, amniotic fluid emboli, infection
■ **14–17wk:** Ultrasound identifies fetal parts and pockets of amniotic fluid
■ **Second half of pregnancy:** Nonstress test to assess fetal well-being
■ **Nursing:**
■ Obtain consent
■ **14–17wk:** Bladder must be full to raise uterus
■ **Second half of pregnancy:** Empty bladder to ↓confusion with uterus; hip roll to ↓hypotension; assess maternal VS, fetal cardiac activity. Mild cramping is common. Fluid leakage is usually self-limiting. Tell patient to avoid intercourse, heavy lifting, and strenuous activity for 24hr after test. Report ↑temp, persistent cramping, or vaginal discharge. Ensure genetic counseling if appropriate. Provide emotional support

AMNIOTIC FLUID TESTS

■ Tests for amniotic fluid with ruptured membranes
■ **Nitrazine test:** Positive test tape dark blue or gray/green
■ **Fern test:** Fern pattern under microscope
■ **Nursing:** Dorsal lithotomy position; encourage coughing to ↑fluid expulsion; touch nitrazine tape to vaginal secretions; for fern test, use cotton-tipped applicator to collect secretions and draw over glass slide

FETAL FIBRONECTIN (FFN)

■ Swab of vaginal/cervical secretions; 22–31wk; FFN leaks with amniotic sac separation; presence may predict labor onset
■ **Nursing:** Assist with dorsal recumbent or lithotomy position; sample collection is obtained like Pap smear

NONSTRESS TEST (NST)

- After 28wk; Doppler transducer records FHR in relation to movement; tocotransducer records fetal movement as changes in uterine pressure
- **Reactive NST:** 2 accelerations (↑ of 15bpm for 15sec) in 20min and normal baseline FHR; predictive of fetal well-being
- **Nonreactive NST:** Failure to meet reactive criteria over 40min; vibroacoustic stimulus for 1sec may be used to startle fetus and can be repeated 2 times
- **Inconclusive:** Less than 2 accelerations in 20min; accelerations do not meet reactive criteria; inadequate quality recording for interpretation
- **Nursing:** Left lateral position to ↓vena cava compression; transducer and tocodynamometer to abdomen; teach to press event button with fetal movement; observe fetal monitor

CONTRACTION STRESS TEST (CST)

- Contractions stimulated and fetal response monitored; done after nonreactive NST; identifies if fetus can withstand ↓O$_2$ during stress of contraction
- **Negative:** Normal baseline FHR, FHR accelerations with fetal movement, and no late decelerations with 3 contractions in 10min indicates healthy fetus; oxytocin discontinued; IV continued until uterine activity returns to prior status; fetus likely to survive labor if it occurs within 1wk with no maternal/fetal change
- **Positive:** Late decelerations with 50% of contractions indicates fetal compromise; monitor mother/fetus; prepare for labor induction
- **Suspicious:** Late decelerations with less than half the contractions
- **Nursing:** Obtain consent; semi-Fowler's with lateral tilt; Doppler transducer to abdomen; 30min baseline maternal VS and FHR; assist with stimulation; monitor IV and mother for signs and symptoms of preterm labor

FETAL MOVEMENT COUNT

- 28wk fetal movement counted by patient at same time daily; more testing indicated for ≤ 3 fetal movements
- **Nursing:** Teach pt to assume a comfortable position; hands on abdomen; count movements for 1hr

DOPPLER STUDIES (UMBILICAL VESSEL VELOCIMETRY)

- Measures blood flow velocity and direction in uterine/fetal structures
- ↓Umbilical vessel flow seen in IUGR, preeclampsia, eclampsia, and postterm
- **Nursing:** Same as fetal ultrasonography

Potential Problems During Pregnancy

DISSEMINATED INTRAVASCULAR COAGULATION (DIC)

- ↑Clotting in microcirculation; platelets and clotting factors become depleted ← bleeding and thromboemboli in organs
- **S&S:** Bleeding, petechiae, purpura, occult blood, hematuria, hematemesis, shock; ↑PT and ↑PTT, ↓platelet count, Hct and fibrinogen levels; ↑risk for DIC in abruptio placentae
- **Nursing:** Assess for signs and symptoms, VS changes, shock; give O_2, heparin, coagulation

FETAL DEMISE: FETAL DEATH IN UTERO (FDIU)

- After 20th wk and before birth. **Stillbirth:** Birth of dead fetus >20wk gestation or wt ≤350gm
- **S&S of FDIU:** No fetal movement/HR, ↓fundal ht, ↓fetal growth; may spontaneously go into labor within 2wk or may be induced
- **Nursing:** Assess signs and symptoms; encourage expression of feelings; support grieving; support memories (seeing, holding, naming, memory box [pictures, blanket, clothing, ID bands, hair lock]); provide for privacy; ensure that family needs are met; refer to support group

HYPEREMESIS GRAVIDARUM

- Intractable N&V beyond 1st trimester causing F&E and nutritional imbalance
- **S&S:** N&V, ↓wt, FVD, electrolyte and acid/base imbalances, ↑Hct, ketonuria
- **Nursing:** Assess signs and symptoms; NPO until dehydration resolves and 48hr after vomiting stops; dry diet if tolerated, advance to small amounts of alternating fluids and solids; IV fluid replacement; antiemetics

MULTIPLE GESTATION

- Multiple fetuses >2° double ovulation, splitting of fertilized egg, or multiple in vitro implantations
- **S&S:** Excessive fetal activity and uterine size, and ↑wt; multiple FHRs; palpation of 3–4 large fetal parts in uterus
- **Nursing:** Assess VS, fetal growth, signs and symptoms of preterm labor; nonreassuring fetal signs; prepare for cesarean; give oxytocic meds postpartum to prevent hemorrhage because of atony 2° uterine over distention

TROPHOBLASTIC DISEASE

- Abnormal growth of tissue and ↑βhCG; hydatidiform mole
- Risk factors include ovulation stimulation, early teens, ≥40yr
- **S&S:** Uterus large for gestational age; no fetal HR, movement, or palpable parts; HTN, hyperemesis and passage of grapelike substance common; confirmed by ultrasonography; risk for hemorrhage, perforation, and infection

- **Nursing:** Assist with suction curettage; avoid induction due to risk of embolization; measurement of βhCG for 1yr; avoid pregnancy for 1yr to allow assessments for signs and symptoms of choriocarcinoma

ECTOPIC PREGNANCY

- Implantation outside uterus; mid-fallopian tube most common site
- **S&S:** Early signs may be obscure; spotting after 1–2 missed periods; sudden, knifelike right or left lower abdominal pain radiating to shoulder (tube rupture); rigid abdomen; signs and symptoms of shock with obscured hemorrhage
- **Nursing:** Assess signs and symptoms, VS for shock, pain pattern, anxiety; give transfusions and pain meds; give RhoGAM to Rh negative patient if appropriate; prepare for repair/removal of tube

INFECTIONS THAT ARE TERATOGENIC

- **Toxoplasmosis:** Protozoal infection; can cause spontaneous abortion in early pregnancy; transmitted via feces of infected cats and raw meat. **Nursing:** Avoid cat litter; cook meat well
- **Rubella:** Viral infection; teratogenic in 1st trimester; congenital defects in heart, ears, eyes, and brain. **Nursing:** Vaccination ≥3mo before pregnancy or after giving birth; avoid others with rubella
- **Cytomegalovirus (CMV):** Viral infection acquired via respiratory or sexual route; fetus may contract infection through birth canal; can cause retardation, deafness, heart defects, and death of neonate. **Nursing:** Teach to avoid others with flulike infections during pregnancy
- **Genital herpes:** Viral infection causing painful, draining vesicles on external genitalia, vagina, and cervix; fetal and neonatal risk are greater when first outbreak occurs during pregnancy; fatal or permanent CNS damage if neonate is infected during vaginal birth. **Nursing:** During active infection: Use contact precautions, prepare for cesarean birth, separate mother and neonate after birth
- **Human immunodeficiency virus (HIV):** Viral infection; ↑transmission risk with advanced disease and prolonged ruptured membranes; antiviral therapy in 2nd and 3rd trimesters and neonate treatment for 6wk postbirth ↓transmission by 66%. **Nursing:** Encourage prenatal care, taking of all meds to ↓viral load, health promotion to ↓opportunistic infections; referrals for HIV counseling and teaching (especially if acquired via risky behavior)

VENA CAVA SYNDROME (SUPINE HYPOTENSIVE SYNDROME)

- Partial occlusion of vena cava by wt of uterus
- **S&S:** ↑Pulse, ↓BP, N&V, diaphoresis, respiratory distress, nonreassuring fetal signs
- **Nursing:** Position on left side to shift wt of fetus off inferior vena cava; monitor VS, FHR, and S&S of shock. Administer O_2

HYPERTENSIVE DISORDERS

Maternal BP ≥140/90. Risk factors include primipara ↓17yr and ↑35yr, multipara, DM, chronic HTN, multiple fetuses, trophoblastic or kidney disease, ↑nutrition, Rh incompatibility. Onset 12–24wk; subsides 6th wk postpartum. Only cure is birth of neonate

Preeclampsia
- **S&S for mild:** 140/90mm Hg or higher; 1+ proteinuria; upper-body edema; progressive excessive ↑wt
- **S&S for severe:** 2 resting BP readings 6hr apart ≥160/110; 3–4+ proteinuria; massive generalized edema; oliguria; sudden large ↑wt; CNS irritability (headache, blurred vision, hyperreflexia)

Eclampsia
- Seizure in pregnancy not attributable to another cause
- **HELLP syndrome:** Hemolysis of RBCs, Elevated Liver enzymes, Low Platelets; variant of severe preeclampsia; multiorgan failure
- **Nursing:** Assess VS and BP q15min when critical, then 1–4hr. Assess edema (I&O, daily ↑wt), CNS irritability (vision problems, hyperreflexia), proteinuria, fetal status, hematological studies, signs of bleeding/labor. Seizure precautions, quiet environment, limit visitors. ↑Protein in diet, moderate sodium intake, give magnesium sulfate (MgSO₄)
- **S&S MgSO₄ toxicity:** Depressed/absent deep tendon reflexes, R ↓12, drug blood level <8mg/dl (therapeutic range 48-mg/dl). Have calcium gluconate available as antidote for MgSO₄; O₂, if ordered. Provide emotional support. Maintain BR in side-lying position during labor and birth. Be prepared for cesarean. Monitor for 48hr postpartum

INCOMPETENT CERVIX
Premature dilation and effacement of cervix; cervix may be sutured closed (cerclage) usually at 10–14wk gestation. Sutures are removed at 37wk
- **S&S:** Painless contractions, vaginal bleeding 18–28wk; fetal membranes observed through cervix
- **Nursing:** Assess signs and symptoms, nonreassuring fetal signs; BR. Prepare for suturing of cervix (cerclage). **Postop:** Maintain BR 24hr, monitor for ruptured membranes, contractions, vaginal bleeding. Teach to avoid intercourse, lifting, prolonged standing

TERMINATION (ABORTION AND ASSISTED ABORTION)
- Spontaneous or planned expulsion of products of conception. Treatment: Mifepristone (RU 486) 1st 9wk, minisuction 1st 5–7wk, vacuum aspiration 1st 12wk, D&C 12–14wk, saline injection 14–24wk
- **Nursing:** Assess VS, bleeding, expelled products, pain, infection. Assess F&E balance. Support grieving. Administer RhoGAM to Rh negative mothers

Labor and Birth

Stages of Labor

Nursing care common to all stages: Establish trust, answer questions, support parents/coach, use standard precautions. Monitor: Contractions, dilation, engagement and position/presentation, fetal/maternal VS (assess between contractions, normal FHR 120–160), dehydration, edema. Provide fluids per orders; encourage voiding q1–2hr; inform parents/MD of progress. For ↓BP: Turn on side and retake. For pulse ox ↓90%: Provide O_2. Fetal monitoring: See page 53. For ruptured membranes: Assess for prolapsed cord, meconium-stained amniotic fluid indicating fetal compromise, S&S of infection

Stage 1: Begins With Regular Contractions and Ends With Fully Dilated Cervix	
Phase	**Nursing Care**
Latent phase: Mild/moderate contractions; q15–30, 15–30sec long; dilation 0–4cm Mother: Alert, excited, verbalizes concerns, may rest/sleep, uses relaxation techniques	Encourage ambulation/upright position if no ruptured membranes Review breathing and focusing techniques. Offer fluids/food if ordered. Assess fetal presentation and position (Leopold's maneuvers)
Active phase: Moderate/strong contractions; q3–5min, up to 60sec long; dilation 4–7cm; membranes may rupture Mother: Alert, more demanding, anxious, restless, may seek pain relief, uses breathing/focusing techniques	Assist with position changes, hygiene and oral care; provide fluids if ordered. Provide counterpressure to sacrococcygeal area, pillow support and backrubs Offer/explain pain meds ordered Talk through contraction Initiate hydrotherapy if desired Encourage breathing and focusing techniques
Transition phase: Strong contractions; every 1–2min; 45–60sec long; dilation 7–10cm Mother: Restless, agitated. May have sudden N&V and pressure on rectum. Has difficulty following directions and focusing	Stay with patient; accept irritability Use relaxation techniques (e.g., effleurage) between contractions Teach to pant (avoids premature pushing) Provide supportive care for N&V and pain relief as indicated Prepare for birth

Stage 2: Begins When Cervix Is Fully Dilated/Effaced and Ends With Birth of Fetus (Pushing Stage)

Dilation complete; progress determined by descent through birth canal (**fetal station**); strong contractions q2–3min, 60–75sec long; ↑bloody show; fetal head visible (**crowning**)

Mother: Relaxes between but pushes with contractions; may complain of severe pain or burning sensation as perineum distends

Nursing: Perform assessments every 5min, monitor FHR before, during, and after contractions. Note duration, intensity, and frequency of contractions with continuous monitoring device
Assist to position that aids pushing
Assess for crowning; encourage panting during contraction (avoids precipitous birth); bearing down with contractions (promotes birth)
Offer mirror to see birth
Prepare for birth

Stage 3: Begins at Birth of Neonate and Ends With Delivery of Placenta (Placental Stage)

Contractions every 3–4min; placental separation and expulsion; Firming and upward movement of fundus, rush of blood from vagina, lengthening umbilical cord; ↑bleeding as uterus shrinks
May have perineal laceration or prophylactic incision (**episiotomy**)

Nursing: Assess neonate; assess VS, fundal tone and contractions until placental delivery; assist to bear down to deliver placenta; give oxytocic & pain meds as ordered
Keep mother and neonate warm
Promote bonding before eye prophylaxis
Put to breast if desired (skin-to-skin); assess parental reaction

Stage 4: First 4hr After Placental Delivery (Recovery Stage)

↑in BP and slight tachycardia expected
Fundus midline, halfway between umbilicus and symphysis pubis; fundus should remain firm and contracted
Scant/moderate red lochia (**lochia rubra**); expected blood loss 250–500mL

Nursing: Assess q15min for 1hr; VS, position and tone of fundus (2 fingerbreadths below umbilicus), bleeding (<2 pads/hr, no free-flow/clots with fundal massage), perineum (sutures intact, no bulging, slight bruising, no severe pain), bladder (nondistended)
Assess spontaneous voiding (>100mL), if discomfort is tolerable (<3 on 1–10 pain scale)
Provide hygiene

Fetal Heart Rate (FHR) Monitoring

FHR monitoring: Number of fetal heartbeats per min; reflects fetal status and, indirectly, a supportive/nonsupportive uterine environment

Auscultation: Obtainable by Doppler 8–12wk, obtainable by fetoscope 16–20wk

Intrapartum electronic monitoring: Patterns reflect expected and abnormal fetal responses during labor; frequency and duration of contractions and FHR variability. **External monitor:** Ultrasound transducer on abdomen over fetal heart and tocotransducer over uterine fundus. **Internal monitor:** Electrode attached to fetal scalp after rupture of membranes

FETAL HEART RATE PATTERNS

■ **Baseline FHR:** FHR between contractions
■ **Normal FHR:** 120–160bpm (can be ↑for short periods <10min)
■ **Tachycardia:** Sustained FHR >160 for >10min; etiologies: early fetal hypoxia, immaturity, amnionitis, maternal fever, terbutaline (Bretha)
■ **Bradycardia:** Sustained FHR <120 for >10min secondary to late/profound fetal hypoxia, maternal hypotension, prolonged cord compression, drugs, and anesthetics
■ **Accelerations:** ↑FHR 15bpm and duration of 15sec; begins with contraction onset and returns to baseline at end; expected fetal response
■ **Decelerations:** ↓FHR in response to onset, peak or relaxation of contractions or fetal activity
  ■ **Early onset:** Fetal head compression, generally benign. Second stage: If close together, stop patient from pushing until FHR returns to normal. Rule out cephalopelvic disproportion if head is above ischial spines.
  ■ **Variable:** Rapid onset and rapid return with variable relationship to contraction. OK if FHR baseline is acceptable; if it lasts >30sec or recovery to baseline is slow, report to MD. Can indicate possible cord compromise (prolapse, around fetal neck/shoulder, knotted). **If due to cord compression:** Stop or ↓oxytocin, lateral position, O_2, IV fluids, prepare for cesarean if not corrected
  ■ **Late onset:** Starts at height of contraction and returns to baseline after contraction ends; reflects uteroplacental insufficiency

Interventions Associated With Labor

LABOR INDUCTION

■ Ripen cervix: Dinoprostone (ProstinE2, Cervidil), prostaglandin gel (PGE_2), laminaria tents; ↑ contractions once uterus is inducible: amniotomy, oxytocin (Pitocin)
■ **Indications:** Postterm, preeclampsia, eclampsia, intrauterine growth restriction, DM, fetal demise
■ **Contraindications:** Placenta previa, prolapsed cord, transverse fetal lie, active genital herpes, vertical cesarean scar

- **Complications:** Uterine tetany (contractions ↓2min apart or lasting >90sec), nausea, ↓urine output
- **Nursing:** Monitor fetal and maternal response; uterine tetany: D/C oxytocin, left side-lying position, give O_2, prepare for cesarean

AUGMENTATION OF LABOR
- Accelerate labor once it has begun; give oxytocin as ordered
- **Indications:** Prolonged or dysfunctional labor, failure to dilate
- Contraindications, complications, and nursing: same as labor induction

ARTIFICIAL RUPTURE OF MEMBRANES (AROM, AMNIOTOMY)
- **Indications:** Hasten labor, permit internal fetal monitoring
- **Complication:** Risk for infection the longer it takes to give birth
- **Nursing:** Assess FHR, maintain horizontal position, assess for cord prolapse; provide perineal care

FORCEPS AND VACUUM ASSISTED BIRTH
- **Maternal indications:** Prolonged 2nd stage; fatigue; maternal illness
- **Fetal indications:** Nonreassuring FHR
- **Complications:** Vaginal/rectal lacerations, fetal injury
- **Nursing: Forceps**—Monitor FHR to ensure cord is not compressed
- **Nursing: Vacuum**—≥35wk apply soft cup over posterior fontanelle, ↑pressure to 440-600mmHg, gentle traction during pushing (D/C after 3 pulls, 20 min, 3 cup detachments or observed scalp trauma); avoid trapping maternal tissue in cup; teach chignon will resolve in 3-7 days, monitor S&S of complications; give support

CESAREAN BIRTH
- Birth via abdominal incision; low transverse incision most common; vertical incision ↑risk of uterine rupture in future pregnancies
- **Indications:** Stalled labor progress (**dystocia**), repeat cesarean, breech presentation, fetal compromise, active genital herpes, placenta previa, abruptio placentae, cord prolapse, preeclampsia, eclampsia
- **Complications:** Wound infection or dehiscence, hemorrhage, bladder/bowel injury, thrombophlebitis, PE; fetal injury or aspiration
- **Nursing:** Emphasis on healthy neonate and mother; teach about surgery, anesthesia, and recovery; assess for S&S of complications

Labor and Birth: Analgesia and Anesthesia

Obstetrical medications presented in TAB 7—Pharmacology and Medication Administration

EPIDURAL BLOCK/INFUSION
- Injection of anesthetic into epidural space to ↓pain of labor and birth
- **Advantages:** Titratable level, patient is awake; nausea & sedation are minimal; urge to push may be preserved; no headache

- **Disadvantages:** Maternal ↓BP; labor progress & fetal descent may be slowed; less effective pushing in 2nd stage; may cause N&V, pruritus, urinary retention
- **Nursing:**
  - Have patient void before; routinely assess for bladder distention
  - Minimize hypotension by giving 500–1000mL IV fluids 15–30min before placement; maintain side-lying position; alternate sides
  - Assist to side-lying or sitting position and support during insertion; patient must remain still; time insertion between contractions
  - Use an infusion pump; ensure catheter placement remains intact
  - Assess VS before & routinely (q1–2min for 1st 10min & then q5–15min); may cause ↓BP & respiratory depression; follow standing orders if ↓BP occurs: terminate infusion, O_2 by mask, Trendelenburg position, bolus of crystalloid fluid, notify practitioner
  - Maintain continuous electronic fetal monitoring
  - Assess pain control; notify practitioner if breakthrough pain occurs because dose is ↓than therapeutic or integrity of line is altered
  - Assess level of sensation & ability to move feet/legs; recovery takes several hr; 2–person assist with 1st ambulation

LOCAL INFILTRATION

- Insertion of analgesia into perineal tissue; ↓pain of birth and episiotomy
- **Advantages:** Technically uncomplicated; does not alter maternal VS or FHR; minimal complications, patient is awake
- **Disadvantages:** A large volume of agent is needed
- **Nursing:**
  - Assess effectiveness
  - Ensure a thermal injury does not occur if cold application is used to ↓inflammation

SPINAL BLOCK

- Injection of anesthetic into spinal fluid provides anesthesia for cesarean birth & occasionally for vaginal birth with midforceps delivery or vacuum extraction
- **Advantages:** Ease of administration, immediate onset, patient is awake, smaller med volume, less shivering, little placental transfer
- **Disadvantages:** Finite duration, possible severe maternal hypotension & total spinal anesthetic response; may ↓ability to push
- **Nursing:**
  - Treat hypotension by giving 500–1000mL IV fluids 15–30min before block
  - Assist to side-lying or sitting position during insertion; patient must remain still. Time insertion between contractions
  - Insert urinary retention catheter before cesarean birth
  - Assess VS before insertion and routinely thereafter
  - Move patient with caution because of temporary leg paralysis

- **Vaginal birth:** Assist to sitting position for 1–2min after block so that solution migrates toward sacral area before side lying. Maintain continuous electronic fetal monitoring. Encourage bearing down during contractions
- **Cesarean birth:** Assist to supine position, with a left lateral tilt, so that cephalad spread of anesthesia occurs
- **Interventions after birth:** Maintain BR for 6–12hr. Two-person assist with first ambulation. Assess for urinary retention because sensation/control may not return for 8–12hr; catheterize as ordered

GENERAL ANESTHESIA
- Induced unconsciousness; requires tracheal intubation with cuffed endotracheal tube, ventilation, and oxygenation
- **Advantages:** Total pain relief; optimum operating conditions
- **Disadvantages:** Patient is not awake; may cause ↑maternal respirations, vomiting, aspiration, uterine atony; may→fetal depression

Nursing:
- Supine position with left-lateral tilt; insert IV line, administer prophylactic antacid as ordered
- Preoxygenate 3–5min with 100% O_2; maintain cricoid ring pressure to occlude esophagus until practitioner inflates cuff of endotracheal tube
- **When extubated:** Maintain open airway, administer O_2, monitor VS, ECG, pulse oximetry; keep suction and resuscitative equipment readily available

Problems During Labor and Birth

ABRUPTIO PLACENTAE
- Partial, marginal, complete separation of placenta from uterine wall >20th wk and before birth
- **S&S:** Painful vaginal bleeding (concealed bleeding if margins are intact); rigid abdomen; shock; nonreassuring fetal signs

Nursing:
- Assess S&S, VS, FHR, bleeding, pain, uterine activity, I&O; serum studies for DIC, PT, and PTT. Keep patient in bed as ordered
- Maintain BR; give O_2, IVs, blood products as ordered; prepare for cesarean birth

AMNIOTIC FLUID EMBOLISM (AFE)
- Escape of amniotic fluid into mother's circulation→pulmonary embolus; 80% fatal; ↑risk of abruptio placentae and hypertonic labor
- **S&S:** Chest pain, respiratory distress, cyanosis, rapid shock, ↑anxiety, feelings of doom, cardiovascular collapse, coagulopathy

- **Nursing:**
  - Assess S&S of AFE during 3rd and 4th stages of labor; aggressive resuscitation
  - IV fluids, PRBC, and platelets to control coagulopathy

BREECH PRESENTATION

- Fetal presenting part is buttocks, legs, feet, or combination thereof; risk for cord prolapse, fetal hypoxia and injury, maternal injury
- **S&S:** Identified via Leopold's maneuvers, FH tone above umbilicus, meconium without nonreassuring fetal signs, vaginal exam
- **Nursing:**
  - Assess S&S, VS, nonreassuring fetal signs, progress of labor
  - Assess birth canal for cord prolapse when membranes rupture
  - Pain relief for "back labor" (massage, IV meds, regional anesthesia)
  - Set up for both vaginal and cesarean birth; give emotional support
  - Nitroglycerin for rapid uterine relaxation if head becomes trapped

PREMATURE RUPTURE OF MEMBRANES (PROM)

- Ruptured membranes before start of labor
- **S&S:** Fluid leaking from vagina, amniotic fluid confirmed with fern or nitrazine test
- **Nursing:**
  - Establish time of rupture
  - Avoid unnecessary vaginal exams
  - Assess for cord compression, FHR, maternal VS, S&S of infection
  - If at term and no labor within 12–24hr, labor is induced
  - **<37wk:** BR in hospital, prophylactic antibiotics, amnioinfusion of isotonic saline to ↓risk of cord compression may be done

PLACENTA PREVIA

- Placenta in lower uterine segment
- **Low lying:** Placenta in close proximity but not covering os; placenta moves away from os as uterus stretches during 3rd trimester (**migrating placenta**)
- **Marginal:** Edge of placenta extends to os and may extend onto os during dilation
- **Partial:** Os is partially covered by placenta
- **Total:** Placenta completely covers os
- **S&S:** 3rd trimester painless bright red bleeding; soft uterus, anemia; ultrasound confirmation
- **Nursing:**
  - BR; no vaginal exams
  - Monitor VS, FHR, blood loss
  - IVs and transfusions for excessive blood loss as prescribed
  - Betamethasone to ↑fetal lung maturity; prepare for preterm birth or cesarean birth

PRECIPITOUS LABOR AND BIRTH

■ **Birth with** <3hr labor
■ **S&S:** Rapid dilation and fetal descent; history of rapid labor; rapid contractions with ↓relaxation between each; risk for fetal intracranial hemorrhage, anoxia; risk for maternal laceration and hemorrhage
Nursing:
■ Remain with patient
■ Encourage panting with contractions
■ Support and guide fetal head during birth
■ Do not stop birth of fetus

PROLAPSED CORD

■ Umbilical cord below presenting fetal part
■ **S&S:** Prolonged variable decelerations and baseline bradycardia; observation of cord protruding through cervix
Nursing:
■ Gently lift presenting part away from cord, which relieves pressure
■ Provide O₂
■ Elevate patient's hips while on side to ↑placental perfusion
■ Assess FHR
■ Notify MD immediately
■ Prepare for possible cesarean

RUPTURED UTERUS

■ Complete/partial separation of uterine tissue from stress of labor/trauma (e.g., scar of previous cesarean); fetal mortality >80%; maternal mortality 50-75%
■ **S&S:** Silent or dramatic; sudden extreme pain; hypotonic/absent contractions; S&S of shock (↓BP, ↑P, pallor, cool clammy skin); may or may not have nonreassuring fetal signs
Nursing:
■ **Prevention:** Cesarean birth after previous cesarean; preventing/limiting uterine hyperstimulation
■ **After rupture:** Administer O₂; prepare for laparotomy for repair or hysterectomy; blood replacement; emotional support

CEPHALOPELVIC DISPROPORTION (CPD)

■ Fetus larger than pelvic diameters; pelvic inlet and/or pelvic outlet diameter narrowed 2° small, abnormally shaped or deformed maternal pelvis
■ **S&S:** Prolonged or arrested 1st or 2nd stage of labor; impaired fetal descent; measurements indicating small pelvic size
Nursing:
■ Assist with x-ray, ultrasonography to identify pelvic size
■ Assess S&S, nonreassuring fetal signs
■ Prepare for cesarean birth

DYSTOCIA

- Difficult, painful, or prolonged labor due to large fetus, cephalopelvic disproportion, malpresentation, abnormal contractions, multiple fetuses
- **S&S: materna** : Exhaustion, extreme pain, ↑P, contractions with ↑frequency and ↓intensity; weak, inefficient or stopped contractions, cervical trauma. **Fetus**: ↑HR, nonreassuring signs, head molding, caput succedaneum, cephalohematoma, demise
- **Nursing:**
  - Assess S&S, progress of labor, maternal VS, infection, status of fetus
  - Monitor response to oxytocin if prescribed
  - Administer pain relief measures
  - Assist with X-ray, ultrasonography to identify pelvic size
  - Have O_2 and resuscitation equipment nearby

PRETERM LABOR

- Start of labor before EDB
- **S&S:** Contractions between 20–37wk with 2cm dilation and 80% effacement; contractions q10min lasting 30sec or longer
- Risk factors: Multiple gestation, maternal illness with ↑temp, opiate use, bacteriuria, multiple abortions, pyelonephritis, bacterial vaginitis
- **Nursing:**
  - Lateral recumbent position, quiet environment, tocolytic agents to suppress labor, such as ritodrine (Yutopar), terbutaline sulfate (Brethine), $MgSO_4$, indomethacin (Indocin), nifedipine (Procardia)
  - Betamethasone (Celestone) to ↓severity of RDS 24–48hr before if birth appears probable
  - Assess FHR, maternal VS, progress of labor; ↓BP with tocolytics
  - Respiratory depression with $MgSO_4$
  - Tachycardia with terbutaline and ritodrine

Postpartum: First 6wk After Birth

Maternal Changes During Postpartum

Vital signs: T ≤ 100.4°F during first 24hr due to exertion and dehydration; BP returns to baseline; P 50–70bpm for 6–10 days due to ↓blood volume and ↓cardiac effort
Nursing: Assess VS q4–8hr. Focused assessment if ↑T (infection), ↑P, and ↓BP (hemorrhage), ↑BP
Reproductive: Fundus: Intermittent contractions return uterus to prepregnant state (**involution**). 12hr after birth, uterus up to or 1 fingerbreadth (FB) above umbilicus, descends 1FB daily, remains firm and in midline, and is not felt by 7–9 days

Nursing: Assess fundal height, massage uterus if boggy but avoid overstimulation. Give oxytocic med if ordered. Teach multipara and breastfeeding mothers that afterpains may accompany involution. Have patient void if uterus is elevated and deviated to right.

Vaginal discharge: Red 2-3 days (**lochia rubra**), pinkish-brown 3-10 days (**lochia serosa**), whitish-yellow 10-21 days (**lochia alba**)
Nursing: Check lochia for color, amount, clots, and odor. Flush perineum and change peripad after voiding and prn. Teach menstruation returns about 6wk when not breastfeeding and 24wk when breastfeeding. Peripad saturated in 15min is excessive; check under buttocks; assess for S&S of shock.

Perineum: Nursing: Assess for hematoma, hemorrhoids, and episiotomy site for Redness, Ecchymosis, Edema, Discharge, and Approximation (REEDA). Cold applications first 24hr (15min on and 45min off), and then warm sitz baths 2-4/day. Use anesthetic spray or witch hazel pads.

Breasts: Soft first 2 days, engorgement 3rd-5th day due to vasodilation.
Nursing: If breastfeeding, see pages 73 and 74. If nonbreastfeeding, wear supportive bra. Use cool applications, fresh cabbage leaves inside bra. Avoid breast stimulation (warm shower, stroking).

Circulatory: ↑WBC, ↓RBC, and ↓Hgb by 4th day. ↑Fibrinogen and ↑platelets by 1st week; blood volume returns to baseline 3rd week.
Nursing: Monitor WBC, RBC, and Hgb. Encourage early ambulation and ↑fluid intake. Promote rest. Assess for S&S of thrombophlebitis.

Urinary: Diuresis in first 24hr ≥2L urine. ↓Bladder tone, perineal edema, or regional anesthesia may → retention. Full bladder displaces uterus up and to the right → ↓involution.
Nursing: Assess I&O, VS. Call MD if patient has not voided within 6-8hr; catheterize if ordered.

Gastrointestinal: ↑Hunger and thirst. ↑Need for protein and calories to support involution and recovery. Usually no BMs for several days due to ↓food during labor, fear of pain (episiotomy and hemorrhoids), and ↓peristalsis during pregnancy.
Nursing: Provide nutritious diet. Assess BMs. Encourage fluids, fiber, and activity to prevent constipation. Give stool softener, suppository, or enema as ordered.

Integumentary: ↑Diaphoresis in first 24hr. Pigmentation changes (striae, linea nigra, and darkened areolae) begin to fade. Separation of rectus abdominis muscles (diastasis recti) may be evident.
Nursing: Promote hygiene.

Emotional:
■ **Phases of maternal adjustment*:**
■ **Dependent (taking-in):** First 24-48hr. Fatigued but exhilarated, reviews birth process, focuses on self, dependent

- ■ **Dependent-independent (taking-hold):** Starts on 2nd and 3rd day and lasts 10–14 days. Begins care of self and infant; eager to learn, still needs nurturing. May have postpartum blues
- ■ **Interdependent (letting-go):** 3rd to 4th week. Focuses on family as a unit, reasserts relationship with partner and resumes sexual intimacy
- ■ **Stages of transition to fatherhood**:**
  - ■ **Stage 1: Expectations:** Preconception of future
  - ■ **Stage 2: Reality:** Realization that expectations not based on fact. Feelings of sadness, ambivalence, jealousy, frustration; desire to be more involved
  - ■ **Stage 3: Transition to mastery:** Conscious decision to take control and become involved with infant

Nursing care for mother and father: Encourage bonding (eye contact, touching, skin-to-skin contact, rooming-in, infant care). Support adjustment to change in role, self-concept. Assess interactions with infant. Observe for S&S of maternal depression or psychosis (see Tab 5). Notify MD.

Problems During Postpartum Period

CYSTITIS
- ■ Bladder infection
- ■ **S&S:** Pain/burning on urination, fever, frequency, hematuria
- ■ **Nursing:** Assess for S&S, distention, fundal height. Obtain urine C&S, ↑fluids to 3000mL daily, encourage frequent/complete emptying of bladder, administer antibiotics

HEMATOMA
- ■ Collection of blood in connective tissue secondary to episiotomy, primigravidity, or use of forceps
- ■ **S&S:** Perineal/rectal pain/pressure, bulging mass in perineum with discoloration, shock
- ■ **Nursing:** Assess S&S. Apply ice, give analgesics or blood products, catheterize patient. Prepare for surgical ligation or evacuation

POSTPARTUM HEMORRHAGE
- ■ Bleeding secondary to uterine atony, laceration, or inversion of uterus during first 24hr postpartum. May also be due to retained placental fragments after first 24hr of birth
- ■ **S&S:** ≥500mL bleeding
- ■ **Nursing:** Stay with patient. Massage fundus. Monitor bleeding (pad count), VS, Hgb, and Hct levels, I&O, IV fluids. Prepare to administer oxytocin and blood transfusions

* From Rubin, R. (1961). Basic maternal behavior. *Nursing Outlook* 9, 683–686.
** From Henderson, A., and Brouse, A. (1991). The experiences of new fathers during the first three weeks of life. *J of Adv Nursing*, 16 (3), 293–298

INFECTION

- Reproductive organ infection within 28 days of birth
- **S&S:** ↑Temp, chills, pelvic/abdominal pain/vaginal discharge, ↑WBC
- **Nursing:** Assess S&S, VS, I&O. Enhance comfort, keep warm. Encourage 3L fluid daily and ↑calorie/protein. Administer antibiotics

MASTITIS

- Infection of breast; often occurs 2–3wk after birth when breastfeeding
- **S&S:** Flulike S&S, ↑temp, local heat/swelling and discomfort/pain
- **Nursing:** Assess S&S; apply heat/cold and give analgesics/antibiotics as ordered. Encourage continued lactation or use of breast pump every 4hr. Suggest use of supportive bra. Teach hand/breast hygiene

PULMONARY EMBOLISM

- Blood clot in lungs from uterine/pelvic veins
- **S&S:** Dyspnea, ↑pulse and respiration, crackles, cough, chest pain, hemoptysis, anxiety
- **Nursing:** Assess for hypoxemia, give O₂, ↑HOB. Administer IV fluids, anticoagulants, and streptokinase to dissolve clot as ordered

SUBINVOLUTION

- Delay of uterus to return to normal size or condition
- **S&S:** ↑Or prolonged lochial discharge, excessive bleeding, uterine pain on palpation, large/boggy uterus
- **Nursing:** Assess S&S, VS, bleeding. Perform firm fundal massage; administer oxytocin or methylergonovine (Methergine) and antibiotics as ordered. Prepare for D&C to remove placental fragments

THROMBOPHLEBITIS

- Inflammation and clot formation inside a vessel caused by venous stasis and hypercoagulation; confirmed by Doppler ultrasound
- **S&S:** Pain/tenderness in lower extremity with heat, redness, swelling, positive Homan's sign
- **Nursing:** Assess S&S, PT, PTT. Keep patient on BR and elevate leg. Give analgesics/anticoagulants (generally IV heparin 5–7 days followed by warfarin [Coumadin] for 3mo) as ordered. Apply warm moist heat; do not elicit Homan's sign or rub area (may→emboli). Apply antiembolism stockings before getting OOB. Teach safety related to anticoagulants (e.g., soft toothbrush, electric razor)

The Newborn

Neonatal Resuscitation Triangle

NEONATAL RESUSCITATION TRIANGLE

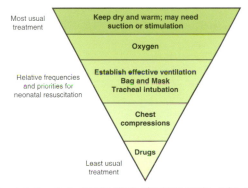

Most usual treatment

Relative frequencies and priorities for neonatal resuscitation

Least usual treatment

Keep dry and warm; may need suction or stimulation

Oxygen

Establish effective ventilation
Bag and Mask
Tracheal intubation

Chest compressions

Drugs

First period of reactivity: First 30–60min after birth; awake, active, strong sucking reflex; HR may >160–180min and irregular. Respirations may >80min, with transient nasal flaring and grunting. No bowel sounds. *Nursing:* Encourage parent-newborn interaction (e.g., eye-to-eye contact, touching, talking, rocking, singing) during first 30–60min. Encourage breastfeeding if desired; provide privacy

Period of inactivity to sleep phase: About 30–60min after birth, newborn's activity↓. Heart rate and respirations gradually↓ to baseline. Sleeps 30min to 4hr; difficult to awaken; no interest in sucking; bowel sounds audible. *Nursing:* Continue close observation

Second period of reactivity: Awakens and is alert; lasts 4–6hr. ↑Response to stimuli. May have ↑respirations and ↑ HR, apneic episodes, mild cyanosis, mottling. May gag, choke, and regurgitate. May pass meconium stool and first void. Sucking, rooting, swallowing indicates readiness for feeding. *Nursing:* Maintain airway; stimulate during apneic episodes. Encourage breastfeeding if desired by mother; document first void and meconium stool

Normal and Abnormal Characteristics of the Neonate

Weight, Length, Gestational Age

Expected Characteristics	Variations/Abnormalities
Term: Birth 37–42wk gestation	**Intrauterine growth restriction (IUGR):** Fetal growth rate differs from gestational age
Appropriate for gestational age (AGA): 10th to 90th percentile for gestational age	
Birth weight: 2500–4000gm; loss of 10% in first wk; regained in 10–14 days	**Preterm:** Birth at <37wk gestation
	Postterm: Birth >42wk gestation
Crown-to-rump length: 31–35cm; circumference approximately equal to chest circumference	**Small for gestational age (SGA):** wt <10th percentile for gestational age
Head-to-heel length: 48–53cm	**Large for gestational age (LGA):** wt >90th percentile for gestational age
Head circumference: 33–35cm	**Low birth weight (LBW):** wt ≤2500gm at birth
Chest circumference: 30.5–33cm	**Very low birth weight (VLBW):** wt ≤1500gm at birth

Vital Signs

Expected Characteristics	Variations/Abnormalities
Axillary temp (T): 97.7°–98.9°F	**Temp:** Hyperthermia, hypothermia
Apical pulse: 100–180bpm after birth and 120–140 when stabilized; murmurs may reflect incomplete closure of fetal shunts	**Pulse:** *Tachycardia:* >160–180bpm; *bradycardia:* <80–100bpm; irregular rhythm; *sinus arrhythmia:* heart rate ↑ on inspiration and ↓ on expiration
Respirations: 30–60bpm, shallow, irregular abdominal; bilateral bronchial breath sounds	**Respirations:** *Tachypnea:* >60bpm; *apnea:* absence of breathing >20sec. Nasal flaring, retractions, diminished breath sounds, expiratory grunting, inspiratory stridor; wheezing, crackles
Blood pressure: oscillometric— 65/41mmHg in arm and calf at 1–3 days of age	**Blood pressure:** Oscillometric systolic pressure in calf 6–9mmHg < pressure in arm may be sign of coarctation of aorta
Preterm: ↑Respiratory effort may require O_2 and ventilation; ↑brown fat and subcutaneous tissue ← temperature instability	

Normal and Abnormal Characteristics of the Neonate *(Continued)*

Skin

Expected Characteristics	Variations/Abnormalities
Bright red, puffy, smooth skin becomes pink, flaky, and dry by 3rd day	Ecchymoses and petechiae
Grayish-white, cheesy deposit covering skin (**vernix caseosa**)	Generalized cyanosis, pallor, mottling, grayness
Fine, downy hair on shoulders, back, and face (**lanugo**). Amount ↓as gestational age↑	When lying on side, lower half of body becomes pink and upper half is pale (**harlequin color change**)
Cyanosis of hands and feet (**acrocyanosis**)	Progressive jaundice, especially during first 24hr usually due to Rh or ABO incompatibility
Transient mottling (**cutis marmorata**) due to stress, overstimulation, cool environment	Tenting of skin (↓skin turgor)
Neonatal jaundice after first 24hr (**physiological jaundice, icterus neonatorum**)	Light brown spots (**café-au-lait spots**)
Preterm: Wrinkled and translucent; abundant lanugo, eyebrows absent, extensive vernix	Port-wine stain (**nevus flammeus**)
Postterm: Dry, cracking, parchmentlike skin without vernix or lanugo. Greenish-tinged skin due to meconium staining	Strawberry mark (**nevus vasculosus**)
	Tiny white papules on cheeks, chin, and nose (**milia**)
	Flat, deep pink localized areas usually on back of neck (**telangiectatic nevi, stork bites**)
	Irregular areas of deep blue pigmentation usually in sacral or gluteal areas (**mongolian spots**)

Posture

Expected Characteristics	Variations/Abnormalities
Slight flexion of extremities	Limp extended extremities, marked head lag (**hypotonia**)
Holds head erect momentarily, turns head from side to side when prone. May have brief tremors	Tremors, twitches, startles easily, arms and hands flexed, legs extended (**hypertonia**)
Preterm: Limp extended limbs, legs abducted	Asymmetric or opisthotonic posturing

(Continued text on following page)

Normal and Abnormal Characteristics of the Neonate (Continued)

Head Shape and Circumference

Expected Characteristics	Variations/Abnormalities
Circumference: see p. 64 Anterior fontanel: Diamond-shaped 1–1.75in Posterior fontanel: Triangle-shaped 0.2–0.4in Fontanels are flat, soft, and firm; bulge when crying Symmetry of face as neonate cries **Preterm:** Head large compared to chest; small fontanels; hair like matted wool; **intracranial hemorrhage:** muscle twitching, seizures, cyanosis, breathing abnormal, shrill cry **Postterm:** Hair may be perfuse	Molding may occur with vaginal birth; head circumference <10th percentile (may indicate **microcephaly**) or >90th percentile (may indicate **hydrocephalus**) Bulging or depressed fontanels when quiet Widened sutures or fontanels; fused sutures Asymmetry of face as neonate cries Diffuse edema of soft scalp tissue that crosses suture line (**caput succedaneum**) Hematoma between periosteum and skull bone (**cephalhematoma**); unilateral and does not cross suture line

Eyes

Expected Characteristics	Variations/Abnormalities
Lids edematous Absence of tears Blink, corneal, and papillary reflexes present Funduscopic examination reveals red reflex Undeveloped fixation on objects Epicanthal folds in neonates of Asian descent	Absence of reflexes Purulent discharge Epicanthal folds in non-Asians Unable to follow bright light Unable to close 1 eye with drawing of mouth to 1 side and inability to wrinkle forehead (**facial palsy**) due to trauma to 7th cranial nerve with vaginal birth or use of forceps

Ears

Expected Characteristics	Variations/Abnormalities
Startle reflex with loud noises Ear cartilages formed, pinna flexible; top of pinna on horizontal line with outer canthus of eye **Preterm:** Ear cartilages undeveloped, ear may fold easily	Low placement Absence of startle reflex in response to noise

Normal and Abnormal Characteristics of the Neonate *(Continued)*

Nose

Expected Characteristics	Variations/Abnormalities
Compressed and bruised Nostrils patent with thin white discharge; sneezing	Nonpatent nostrils Purulent or copious nasal discharge Flaring of nares

Mouth

Expected Characteristics	Variations/Abnormalities
Intact, arched palate with uvula in midline Frenulum of tongue and upper lip Extrusion, gag, rooting, and sucking reflexes present Minimal salivation Vigorous cry	Incomplete closure of lip (**cleft lip**); incomplete closure of plate or roof of mouth (**cleft palate**) Enlarged, protruding tongue; profuse salivation Cry: Absent, weak, high-pitched White patches on oral membranes and tongue (**candidiasis, thrush**)

Neck

Expected Characteristics	Variations/Abnormalities
Short, thick with multiple skin folds Tonic neck reflex present	Excessive skin folds; absence of tonic neck reflex

Chest

Expected Characteristics	Variations/Abnormalities
Anteroposterior and lateral diameters equal Xiphoid process evident Bilateral areola and breast bud tissue 0.5–1.0cm; breast tissue ↑as gestational age↑ Mild sternal retractions on inspiration **Preterm:** Absent or ↓breast tissue	Depressed sternum, funnel chest (**pectus excavatum**), pigeon chest (**pectus carinatum**) Wide-spaced nipples, extra nipples (**supernumerary nipples**) Milky discharge from breast (**"witch's milk"**) Marked retractions during inspiration Asymmetric chest expansion

(Continued text on following page)

Normal and Abnormal Characteristics of the Neonate (Continued)

Abdomen

Expected Characteristics	Variations/Abnormalities
Umbilical cord: Bluish-white; 2 arteries and 1 vein Presence of bowel sounds Liver: Palpable 2–3cm below right costal margin Spleen: Tip palpable left costal margin Kidneys: Palpable 1–2cm above umbilicus by 1wk Preterm: ↓Bowel sounds	Presence of 1 artery in cord Umbilical hernia obvious when crying Cord bleeding or hematoma Gap between rectus muscles (diastasis recti) Abdominal distention; absent bowel sounds Visible peristaltic waves Enlarged liver or spleen

Back and Rectum

Expected Characteristics	Variations/Abnormalities
Spine intact Trunk incurvation (Galant) reflex present Patent anal opening Passage of meconium within 24hr Anal constriction when touched (anal wink)	External saclike protrusion along spinal column (spina bifida) Dimple with tuft of hair along spine (pilonidal cyst); may indicate underlying spina bifida occulta No trunk incurvation (Galant) reflex Imperforate anus No meconium passed within 36hr

Extremities

Expected Characteristics	Variations/Abnormalities
Symmetrical with full ROM; 10 fingers and toes. Feet flat, creases on anterior 2/3 of sole Preterm: Fine wrinkles; flexing of hand toward forearm creates angle that ↓with ↑in gestational age (square window sign) Elbow in relation to midline when arm is drawn across chest: The farther the elbow passes the midline, the ↑gestational age (scarf sign) Postterm: Long fingernails	Extra digits, fused/webbed digits, palmar simian crease ↑ROM, fractures of clavicle, humerus, or femur. Signs of paralysis Audible click on flexion and abduction of hips (Ortolani's sign); unequal gluteal or leg folds. May indicate developmental dysplasia of the hip Fixed plantar flexion with medial deviation (clubfoot, talipes equinovarus) Flaccid arm with elbow extended and hand internally rotated (Duchenne-Erb paralysis) due to birth trauma

Normal and Abnormal Characteristics of the Neonate *(Continued)*

Male Genitalia

Expected Characteristics	Variations/Abnormalities
Urethral opening at tip of penis Scrotum developed (pendulous, multiple rugae, and contains testes) May be unable to retract foreskin Urination within 24hr **Preterm:** Scrotum undeveloped	Urethra opens on ventral surface (**hypospadias**) or dorsal surface (**epispadias**) Ventral curvature of penis (**chordee**) Fluid in scrotum (**hydrocele**) Testes not palpable Ambiguous genitalia No urination within 24hr

Female Genitalia

Expected Characteristics	Variations/Abnormalities
Urethral opening between clitoris and vagina Labia majora developed; nonprominent clitoris Urination within 24hr **Preterm:** Labia majora incompletely developed, clitoris prominent	Enlarged clitoris with urethral opening at tip Fused labia, no vaginal opening Blood-tinged or mucoid vaginal discharge (**pseudomenstruation**) Ambiguous genitalia No urination within 24hr

Assessment of the Newborn

		Apgar Score		Assessments	
		Possible Scores			
Sign	0	1	2	1Min	5Min
Respiratory effort	Absent	Slow, irregular, weak cry	Strong loud cry		
Heart rate/pulse	Absent	<100bpm	>100bpm		
Muscle tone/activity	Flaccid	Limited movement, some flexion of extremities	Active movement		
Reflex irritability	None	Grimace, limited cry	Vigorous cry		
Color/appearance	Pale, blue	Pink torso, blue extremities	Pink torso & extremities		
Total Score					

Rating total scores: Normal 7–10   4–6 Moderate Depression   0–3 Aggressive Resuscitation

Reflexes in the Neonate

Reflex Name	Physical Response
Babinski	When stimulating outer sole of foot from heel upward and across ball of foot toward large toe, large toe dorsiflexes and toes flare; persists 1yr
Blink	When startled or quick movement is made toward eye, eyelids close; persists for life
Corneal	When cornea is directly stimulated, eyelids close; persists for life
Crawl	When placed on abdomen, arms and legs make crawling motions; persists 6wk
Extrusion	When tongue is touched, tongue moves forward out through the lips; persists 4mo
Gag	When stimulating posterior pharynx, choking occurs; persists for life
Grasp	When palm (palmar reflex) or sole of foot (plantar reflex) is stimulated at base of digits, fingers/toes flex in griplike motion; persists 3 and 8mo, respectively
Moro (startle)	When startled (noise, jarring), arms extend and abduct with fingers forming a C while knees and hips flex slightly, arms return to chest in an embracing motion; persists 3–4mo
Step (dance)	When supported under both arms with feet against firm surface, feet will make stepping movements; persists 3–4wk
Pupillary	When retina stimulated by light, pupil constricts; persists for life
Rooting	When touching cheek or lips, head turns toward touch and mouth opens in attempt to suck; lasts 3–4mo, may persist 1yr
Sucking	When object touches lips or is placed in mouth, sucking is attempted; persists through infancy
Tonic neck (fencing)	When supine with head turned to one side, extremities on same side straighten and extremities on opposite side flex; persists 3–4mo
Trunk incurvation (Galant)	When stroking infant's back alongside spine, hips move toward stimulated side; persists 4wk

Nursing Care of the Newborn

Identification: Apply matching ID bracelets to newborn and mother with name, sex, date, and time of birth. ID number (significant others may also wear bracelets). Obtain newborn footprint on form with mother's fingerprints, name, date, and time of birth. Identify before mother and newborn are separated.

Patent airway: Suction mouth and then nasal passages. Insert bulb syringe or Delee catheter along side of mouth to avoid gag reflex; use side-lying position with roll behind back.

Body temperature: Dry baby thoroughly, put on a cap, place on mother's abdomen. Cover with warm blanket in an isolette or unclothed under radiant warmer. Assess temperature (use axillary or thermoprobe) q1h until stable. Rectal temp route contraindicated. Newborn is unable to shiver and breaks down brown fat to produce energy for warmth. Stress ↑ need for O₂ and upsets acid-base balance.

Eye prophylaxis: Insert ophthalmic antibiotic (e.g., 0.5% erythromycin, 1% tetracycline) into lower conjunctiva of each eye—prevents gonorrheal or chlamydial infection of eyes **(ophthalmia neonatorum)** contracted during vaginal birth. Insert after parent-newborn attachment is facilitated.

Vitamin K: Administer IM dose of vitamin K (0.5–1.0mg phytonadione) to promote normal clotting. Vitamin K is produced in the GI tract when bacterial formation occurs after ingesting breast milk or formula, usually by 8th day.

Umbilical cord: Clamp for 24hr until cord is dry. Assess for bleeding or infection. Clean cord with soap and water after each diaper change and apply topical antibiotic if ordered. Place diaper below umbilical cord stump. Continue care until cord falls off (about 10–14 days).

Bathing: Bathe with warm water and mild soap to remove amniotic fluid, blood, vaginal secretions, and skin residue. Keep environment warm and draft-free to ↓chilling. Dry and swaddle baby. Sponge bathe daily—tub bath after cord falls off and circumcision is healed (usually 2wk).

Circumcision: Assess for swelling, redness, bleeding q30min for 2hr, then q2h for 24hr, then with each diaper change. Monitor urination (<6 diapers a day may indicate urethral edema is occluding urethra). Change dressing as ordered (e.g., 3 times on first day and then daily for 3 days. Use A&D ointment or petroleum jelly). Avoid disrupting yellowish exudate that appears on second day, as this is part of the healing process. Apply diaper loosely to ↓pressure and friction. Give analgesic as ordered.

Breastfeeding

MATERNAL BENEFITS

Increases attachment. Releases oxytocin promoting uterine contraction and involution (lochia flow may ↑). Energy and calories ↑wt reduction. Extends anovulation beyond 4–6wk (contraception should be discussed with MD if desired). Convenient and economical; ↓risk of breast and ovarian cancer

NEWBORN BENEFITS

Increases attachment; optimum nutritional value for 1st 6mo of age (vitamin D and fluoride supplements should be given after 6mo); provides immunological components (passive immunity via IgE, IgM, and IgA immunoglobulins, macrophages, leukocytes, lymphocytes, neutrophils); ↓incidence of morbidity and mortality

CONTRAINDICATIONS

Mother: HIV positive, active TB, narcotic addiction, breast abnormalities from trauma, burns, radiation. Chronic disease that interferes with lactation or maternal status. Taking drugs excreted in breast milk that are harmful to infant. Inadequate maternal fluid/nutrition intake

Newborn: Anomalies that prevent ingestion (e.g., cleft palate) or inborn errors of metabolism that cause negative response to breast milk. Preterm infant may not have energy to suck; breast milk may be given by bottle or gastric tube.

Nursing Care Related to Breastfeeding

- Document mother's desire to breastfeed, level of anxiety, family support, knowledge and demonstration of effective breast care and breastfeeding, condition of nipples, and maternal and infant response.

TEACH SELF-BREAST CARE

- Cleanse breasts with water daily (soap and alcohol cause drying)
- Wear a supportive brassiere day and night
- Wear nursing pads to absorb leaking milk; allow nipples to air-dry several times a day.

TEACH BREASTFEEDING TECHNIQUES

- Begin breastfeeding as soon as possible (preferably in birthing room)
- Offer breast q2–3hr or on demand (feeding cues include sucking movements, hand-to-mouth motions)
- Assume comfortable position (semireclining, sitting); place infant with entire body facing breast (cradle, side-lying, football hold)
- Alternate starting breast and use both breasts at each feeding (↑milk production)

■ Stimulate rooting reflex and direct nipple and entire areola into open mouth above tongue (**latching-on**). Nipple stimulation or emotional response to infant precipitates tingling sensation in breast as milk enters ducts and is secreted from breasts (**let-down reflex**)

■ Burp infant during and after feeding—rub or pat back while infant sits on mother's lap, flexed forward (allows monitoring of airway)

■ Place infant on side with back roll or supine after feeding (↑regurgitation and SIDS)

■ Breast milk may be pumped and stored for future use. Refrigerate for 72hr or freeze for ≤6mo. Date each bottle and use oldest first.

Problems Encountered With Breastfeeding

BREAST ENGORGEMENT

■ Breasts are swollen, hard, hot, tender, and may be dry and red due to vascular congestion before secreting milk (**lactation**); usually occurs 3–5 days postpartum

■ **Nursing:**
■ Breastfeed q2h and empty breasts entirely by pumping (back pressure on full milk glands ↑milk production)

■ Apply ice between feedings 15min on and 45min off (heat ↑vascular congestion)

INVERTED NIPPLES

■ Nipples are below surface of surrounding skin

■ **Nursing:**
■ Wear breast shield to draw nipple out
■ Use electric breast pump before attempting latching-on
■ Apply ice and tug and roll nipple with hands before feeding

SORE OR CRACKED NIPPLES

■ Nipple irritation resulting in discomfort

■ **Nursing:**
■ Alternate infant position
■ Ensure infant is on areola and not just the nipple
■ Apply ice before feeding to ↑nipple erectness and ↓soreness OR breast massage and warm compress before feeding to ↑let-down reflex
■ Analgesic 1hr before feeding to ↓soreness
■ Use less sore nipple first
■ Use breast shield. At end of feeding apply breast milk to nipples and air-dry

Formula Feeding (Bottle-Feeding)

BENEFITS
More freedom for mother; permits feeding by significant others. Allows for accurate assessment of intake. Special formulas can be given for infants with allergies or inborn errors of metabolism. Appropriate for infants with congenital anomalies (e.g., cleft palate)
CONTRAINDICATIONS
Cost of formula/equipment. Lack of time or ability to prepare/store/refrigerate bottles of formula. Potential for contaminated water supply

Nursing Care Related to Formula Feeding

TEACH FORMULA AND FORMULA PREPARATION
- Formula should yield 110–130 calories and 130–200mL of fluid/kg of body weight
- From birth to 2mo 6–8 feedings of 2–4oz of formula may be ingested in 24hr
- Formula may be ready-to-feed, concentrated, or powder; 1 day's supply at a time should be prepared
- Sterilization may be necessary if water source is questionable
- Regular cow's milk not appropriate <12mo of age because of ↑protein and ↑calcium and less vitamin C, iron, and CHO than breast milk

TEACH FORMULA-FEEDING TECHNIQUES
- Warm bottle by placing it in warm water (never use microwave oven)
- Sprinkle a few drops on wrist to test temperature
- Offer bottle every $2^1/_2$-4hr or on demand
- Start with 3oz in each bottle
- Always hold infant (propping bottle may cause aspiration)
- Support entire length of body with head elevated and attempt eye-to-eye contact; keep nipple filled with formula (↓air ingestion)
- Adjust nipple hole size (e.g., infant with ↓sucking reflex or ↓energy requires bigger hole)
- Burp during and after feeding
- Place infant on side with back roll after feeding (↓regurgitation)
- Discard unused formula

PROBLEMS ENCOUNTERED WITH FORMULA FEEDING
- Overdilution of formula →inadequate ↑wt
- Underdilution of formula →excess ↑wt
- Infant may not tolerate fats or CHO found in formula
- Bacterial contamination during preparation and storage may occur

Vital Sign Ranges

Age-Appropriate Vital Signs

	Heart Rate	Respirations	Blood Pressure
Newborn	80–180	30–60	60–80/30–60
Toddler	90–110	24–32	90–100/55–65
School Age	60–110	18–26	95–110/55–70
Adolescent	50–90	16–20	80–120/50–80
Adult	60–100	12–20	110–140/60–90

Immunization Schedule—United States 2007

Hepatitis B (HepB): 1st dose after birth before discharge, 2nd at 4wk after 1st dose, 3rd at ≥24wk. IM

Diphtheria, tetanus, pertussis (DTaP): dose at 2, 4, 6mo, 4th at 15–18mo, 5th at 24–6yr; tetanus and diphtheria toxoids (Tdap) recommended at 11–12yr and boosters every 10 yr. IM

Haemophilus influenzae b (Hib) conjugate vaccine: dose at 2 and 4mo. IM

Inactivated polio (IVP): dose at 2 and 4mo, 3rd at 6–18mo, 4th at 4–6yr. Sub-Q

Measles, mumps, and rubella (MMR): 1st dose at 12–15mo, 2nd at 4–6yr. Sub-Q

Varicella (VAR): 1st dose 12–15 mo, 2nd at 4–6yr. IM or Sub-Q

Pneumococcal (PVC): dose at 2, 4, 6mo, 4th dose at ≥12mo. IM or Sub-Q

Influenza: 1st dose at 6mo; yearly ≥59mo. IM

Hepatitis A: 2 doses 6mo apart between 12–24 mo. IM

Human papillomavirus 2: 3 doses, 11–12yr, 2nd 2mo after 1st dose, 3rd 4mo after 2nd dose. IM

Rotavirus vaccine (Rota): 3 doses, 2, 4, 6mo. Do not initiate ≥12wks, final dose given before 32wk. Oral

NURSING CARE FOR CHILDREN RECEIVING AN IMMUNIZATION

■ Contraindications: High fever, acquired passive immunity (maternal antibodies, blood transfusions, immunoglobulin), immunosuppression, previous allergic response, pregnancy—MMR.

■ Follow schedule

■ Local reactions—use appropriate-length needle to reach muscle

■ Use age-appropriate muscle—vastus lateralis or ventrogluteal for infants, deltoid may be used ≥18mo

- Apply topical anesthetic spray at injection site. Inject slowly
- Teach side effects: *Systemic*—low-grade T; *local*—tenderness, erythema, and swelling; *behavioral*—drowsiness, irritability, anorexia

Growth and Development

Infant: 1–12 Months

PHYSICAL

- Weight triples; chest approaches head circumference; 6–8 teeth
- Turns from abdomen to back by 5mo and back to abdomen by 6mo
- Sits by 7mo. Crawls, pulls self up, and uses pincer grasp by 9mo
- Walks holding on by 11mo

PSYCHOSOCIAL

- Task is development of trust that →faith and optimism; support task by meeting needs immediately
- Oral stage—provide pacifier for comfort and to meet oral needs
- Egocentric; smiles and focuses on bright objects by 2mo. Laughs by 4mo. Separation anxiety begins by 4–8mo. Fears strangers by 6–8mo—provide consistent caregiver
- May have "security object"—keep object available

COGNITIVE

- Sensorimotor phase; reflexes replaced by voluntary activity
- Beginning understanding of cause/effect by 1–4mo
- Realizes objects moved out of sight still exist (**object permanence**) by 9–10mo

LANGUAGE

- Crying signals displeasure first 6mo
- Babbles by 3mo; imitates sounds by 6mo; reacts to simple commands by 9mo; says 1 word by 10mo; says 3–5 words and understands 100 by 12mo

PLAY

- Plays alone (**solitary**); involves own body; becomes more interactive and shows toy preferences by 3–6mo; involves sensorimotor skills by 6–12mo—ensure play is interactive, recreational, and educational
- **Toys:** Must be large enough to prevent aspiration; should be simple secondary to short attention span. Black/white or bright mobiles, stuffed animals, rattles, teething rings, push-pull toys, blocks, books with textures

Toddler: 12–36 Months

PHYSICAL

- ↓Growth rate; birth weight quadruples by 2.5yr
- Anterior fontanel closed by 18mo; chest >head circumference
- ↓Appetite (**physiological anorexia**); 20 teeth
- ↑Naps; daytime bowel/bladder control at 2yr and night control by 3–4yr
- ↑Taste preferences; walks by 14mo; runs by 18mo
- Mastery of gross and fine motor movements

PSYCHOSOCIAL

- Task is autonomy ← self-control—encourage independence
- Anal stage of development
- Notes sex role differences and explores own body
- Differentiates self from others
- Withstands short periods of delayed gratification and parental separation

INJURY PREVENTION

- *Suffocation/aspiration:* Avoid pillows, excessive bedding, tucked-in blankets, baby powder, propping bottles, latex balloons, buttons, plastic bags, crib slats >2³/₂ inch, blind cords, hot dogs, grapes, nuts, raisins
- *Motor vehicle injuries:* Use rear-facing car seat with 5-point harness; do not leave in car unattended
- *Falls:* Supervise when on raised surface; place gates at top/bottom of stairs; use restraints with infant seat, high chair, walker, or swing
- *Poisoning:* Store agents in high/locked cabinet; avoid secondhand smoke; keep poison control center number by telephone
- *Burns:* Set water heater at 120°F, test water before bath, use bathtub not sink for baths, avoid exposure to sun, do not use microwave to warm bottle; put inserts in electric outlets and smoke/heat detectors throughout house
- *Drowning:* Supervise when in/near water such as bathtub, toilet, bucket, pool, lake; keep toilet lid down

REACTION TO ILLNESS, HOSPITALIZATION, AND PAIN

- Before 6mo recognizes pain but is not emotionally traumatized by intrusive procedures
- **S&S of pain:** ↑Pitched cry, irritability, tearing, stiff posture, fisting, brows lowered and drawn together, eyes tightly closed, mouth open, difficulty sleeping/eating
- **Nursing:** Meet needs immediately to ↑ trust. Provide nipple dipped in sucrose solution during painful procedure; give ordered meds. After 6mo see information under Toddler

- Negativistic—give choices, avoid frustration, provide for safety while ignoring tantrum
- Needs routines and may suck thumb for comfort—support routines
- May have a "security object"
- May fear sleep, engines, animals
- Sibling rivalry with newborn—supervise interaction, give individual attention, and include in newborn care, provide doll for imitative play

COGNITIVE

- Continuation of sensorimotor phase
- Preconceptional thought by 2–4yr; beginning of memory
- ↑Sense of time; asking "why" and "how" by 2yr; magical thinking
- ↑Concept of ownership ("mine"); beginning conscience

LANGUAGE

- ↑Comprehension; 4–6 words/15mo, ≥10/18mo, and >300/2yr
- Talks incessantly; sentences by 2yr

PLAY

- Plays alongside, not with, other children (**parallel play**), imitative
- Types of play: Interactive, recreational, and educational
- Interactions: Alone, peers, adults
- Environments: Home, park, preschool; activities: quiet, active, structured, unstructured (provide varieties of play)
- **Toys:** *Physical*—push-pull, pounding board, pedal-propelled, balls. *Social/creative*—telephone, dolls, safe kitchen utensils, dress-up, trucks. *Fine motor skills*—crayons, nesting blocks; tactile—finger paints, clay. *Cognitive*—simple puzzles, picture books, appropriate TV/videos

INJURY PREVENTION

- *Motor vehicle:* Use rear-facing seat at <20lb and forward-facing seat at 20–40lb. Special restraints used until 60lb or 8yr
- *Drowning:* Supervise when in/near water. Fence/cover pool/hot tub. Know CPR
- *Burns:* Turn handles of pots to back of stove; front guards on radiators, space heaters, fireplaces; keep appliance cords, candles, and irons out of reach
- *Poisoning:* Same as infant
- *Suffocation/aspiration:* Avoid foods that may occlude airway (nuts, grapes, hot dogs, hard candy). Keep garage door openers inaccessible. Avoid toy boxes with heavy hinged lids, clothing with drawstrings, and appliances that cannot be opened from inside
- *Bodily damage:* Do not run with objects in mouth, hold pointed objects downward, or run/jump near glass doors. Keep tools and firearms in locked cabinet. Keep away from lawnmowers. Never go with a stranger or allow inappropriate touching

Preschooler: 3–5 Years

PHYSICAL
- Average ↓weight 5lb/yr and ↑height 2.5–3in/yr
- ↑Immune responses
- ↑Strength
- Refinement of gross/fine motor skills
- Dresses and washes self
- Skips, hops, jumps rope, skates, holds pencil and utensils with fingers, and uses scissors by 5yr
- Potential for amblyopia by 4–6yr—assess for nonbinocular vision (strabismus)

PSYCHOSOCIAL
- Task is development of initiative → direction and purpose encourage endeavors
- Oedipal stage of psychosexual development; attaches to parent of opposite sex while identifying with same-sex parent—encourage imitative and imaginative play; begin informal sex education
- May have imaginary friend
- Selfish, impatient, and exaggerates
- Beginning morality (right/wrong)
- Personality developed by 5yr

COGNITIVE
- ↑Preconceptual thought; intuitive thought by 4–5yr
- ↑Readiness for learning; curious about immediate world
- Considers another's views; understands past, present, future by 5yr

REACTION TO HOSPITALIZATION, ILLNESS, AND PAIN
- Fears punishment, the unknown, and separation
- Immobilization, isolation, and altered rituals ↑stress. Regresses when anxious
- Stages of separation anxiety:
  - Protest: Inconsolable crying and rejects others
  - Despair: Flat affect, unresponsive to stimuli, altered sleep, ↓appetite
  - Detachment/denial: Lack of preference for parents, friendly to all
- **S&S of pain:** Expresses pain in a word ("ow"); regresses; clings to parent; cries
- **Nursing:** Provide consistency; ignore regression while praising appropriate behavior; provide consistent caregiver; stay with child, provide massage, distraction, meds, and thermotherapy as ordered

LANGUAGE

- ↑Complexity. Uses all parts of speech, asks the meaning of new words
- Knows 900 words by 3yr, 1500 by 4yr, and 2100 by 5yr
- Stuttering and stammering common during 2–4yr

PLAY

- Group play without rigid rules (**associative play**)
- Physical, manipulative, imitative, and imaginary play
- ↑Sharing by 5yr
- **Toys:** *Physical*—playground and sports equipment, bicycles. S*ocial and creative*—dress-up, puppets, villages. *Fine motor skills*—construction sets, musical instruments, craft projects. *Cognitive*—educational computer games (numbers, letters), simple board games, activity books

INJURY PREVENTION

- Similar to toddler but not as significant due to ↑fine and gross motor skills, coordination, and balance
- ↑Awareness of danger and parental rules
- Pedestrian/motor vehicle accidents occur because of bicycle riding, running after balls into street, crossing streets—teach safety habits: "Look both ways," wear helmets, and play in yard or playground. Parents should set example of acceptable behavior

REACTION TO ILLNESS, HOSPITALIZATION, AND PAIN

- Fears intrusive procedures, pain, punishment, rejection, bodily harm, castration, and darkness more than separation
- **S&S of pain:** Crying, biting, hitting, kicking
- Death viewed as temporary
- **Nursing:** To ↓anxiety, explain and demonstrate what may be experienced. Visit the hospital, support therapeutic play with dolls and medical equipment. Use distraction, thermotherapy, massage, and meds as ordered

School-Age Child: 6–12 Years

PHYSICAL

- Bone precedes muscular development
- Average ↑height 2in/yr and ↑weight 4.5–6.5lb/yr; girls pass boys in height and weight by 12yr
- Permanent teeth beings with front teeth; puberty begins earlier in females (10yr) than males (12yr)

PSYCHOSOCIAL

- Task is achievement of industry →personal/interpersonal competence—recognize accomplishments, avoid comparisons
- Latent stage of psychosexual development; ↓egocentricity

- Identifies with peers of same sex by 6–10yr; beginning interest in opposite sex by10–12yr
- Develops intrinsic motivation (mastery, self-satisfaction)
- Behaves according to set norms
- Develops self-image and body image

COGNITIVE
- Concrete operations, inductive reasoning, and beginning logic by 7–11yr
- Grasps concepts of conservation
- Classifies, serializes, tells time, and reads

LANGUAGE
- Vocabulary and comprehension expand
- Adult speech well established by 9–12yr

PLAY
- ↑Ego mastery; conformity in play; fanatic about rules
- ↑in peer relationships (team sports, clubs)
- ↑Complexity of board games
- Collections become more selective; hero worship—promote positive role model

INJURY PREVENTION
- ↑Risk-taking behaviors secondary to ↓physical abilities, ↓parental supervision, poor judgment
- More injuries in boys than girls
- *Motor vehicle injuries:* teach pedestrian skills, use backseat, wear seat belt, and play in park not street
- *Bodily damage:* wear eye, mouth, and ear protection with sports; avoid unsupervised gymnastics and climbing; never go with a stranger or allow inappropriate touching
- *Toxic substances:* Role-play saying "no" to tobacco, drugs, and alcohol

REACTION TO ILLNESS, HOSPITALIZATION, AND PAIN
- Fears the unknown, ↓control, dependency, disfigurement, death
- **S&S of pain:** Tries to cooperate or stays rigid for painful procedures but may cry, yell, or resist; clenched fists; gritted teeth; closed eyes; wrinkled forehead; personifies death as "bogeyman" but has realistic concept by 9–10yr
- **Nursing:** Place with age-appropriate roommate, support visits from peers and doing schoolwork. Provide privacy, permit wearing underpants. Allow manipulation of equipment, avoid procrastination, provide choices, praise attempts at cooperation, encourage expression of feelings. Never belittle regression, resistance, or crying. Use pain scale and distraction, guided imagery, thought stopping, soothing music, thermotherapy, massage, meds as ordered

Adolescent (12–21 Years)

Early adolescence (11–14yr): Changes of puberty and reaction to changes
Middle adolescence (15–17yr): Transition to peer group identification
Late adolescence (18–21yr): Transition into adulthood

PHYSICAL

- Uncoordinated as linear exceeds muscular growth; ↑strength, especially males
- **Male puberty:** 12–16yr; enlargement of scrotum, testes, and penis; pubic, axillary, facial, and body hair; nocturnal emissions and mature spermatozoa; voice deepens; 95% of height by 15yr
- **Female puberty:** 10–14yr; breasts develop; pubic and axillary hair; first menstruation (**menarche**); ovulation about 12mo after menarche; 95% of height by menarche

PSYCHOSOCIAL

- Feel omnipotent; behavior motivated by peer group
- ↑Interest in appearance
- Desire independence but may avoid responsibilities
- Resist enforcement of discipline
- ↑Interest in sex (experimentation); form intimate relationships (opposite sex if heterosexual and same sex if homosexual)

COGNITIVE

- Formal operational thought; capable of abstract, conceptual, and hypothetical thinking; comprehend satire, double meanings
- ↑Learning through inference vs. repetition/imitation
- Difficulty accepting another's viewpoint; idealistic
- Develop personal value systems (value autonomy)

LANGUAGE

- ↑Vocabulary and reading comprehension
- Experiment with language; use jargon

PLAY

- Individual and team sports provide exercise, ↑social and personal development, and permit experience of competition, teamwork, and conflict resolution
- Follow rules of complex games (Monopoly, chess)

INJURY PREVENTION

- Risk-taking secondary to feelings of omnipotence, assert independence, or impress peers
- *Motor vehicle:* Assess level of responsibility and ability to resist peer pressure; set limits on driving

- *Sports:* Encourage warming-up and cooling-down, playing within abilities, and wearing protective gear
- *Suicidal/homicide:* Males more than females; related to economic deprivation, family dysfunction, and availability of firearms; Assess risk due to frustration, depression, aggression, social isolation. Lock up firearms. Teach to go to school nurse if experiencing sexual harassment/abuse
- *Sexually transmitted infections (STI):* May not seek medical care due to lack of S&S, misinformation, guilt, shame, fear. Teach sex education and STI prevention (abstinence or ↑number of partners, use of condoms). Role-play resisting peer pressure

REACTION TO ILLNESS, HOSPITALIZATION, AND PAIN
- Similar to school-age child with ↑need for independence, privacy, and body integrity
- Fear of disfigurement or ↓function
- ↓Need for parental visits but separation from peers may be traumatic
- **S&S of pain:** Physical pain tolerated; stoicism important among males; clenched fist/teeth, self-splinting; ↑interest and concentration; has realistic concept of death but emotionally may be unable to accept it
- **Nursing:** Use distraction, music, massage, meds as ordered; encourage peer visits

Common Human Responses

Constipation

ETIOLOGY AND PATHOPHYSIOLOGY
- ≥3 days without BM; painful; blood-streaked BMs; stool retention with or without soiling; long intervals between BMs (**obstipation**)
- **Idiopathic or functional constipation:** Majority of constipation has no organic cause such as transient illness, dietary changes, travel, meds, withholding behaviors associated with painful BMs or overzealous toilet training, emotional stress (lack of privacy)
- More common in formula-fed infants; breast-fed infants may have infrequent BMs because of digestibility of breast milk

SIGNS AND SYMPTOMS
- Distended abd, rectal fullness, straining at stool, blood-streaked BMs, ↓bowel sounds

TREATMENT
- Transient constipation resolves spontaneously
- Mild constipation resolves with intro of solid foods; stool softeners (lactulose); laxatives (MOM, polyethylene glycol [Miralax])
- **Impaction:** Suppositories, enemas, GoLIGHTLY, mineral oil

NURSING

- ■ Rectal stimulation with cotton-tipped applicator or thermometer is contraindicated →pain and anal fissures. Oral mineral oil can be given—administer carefully to prevent aspiration
- ■ Assess: Age at onset; bowel habits; stools for frequency, amount, color, and consistency; diet (breastfeeding, formula feeding, fluids, foods
- ■ Teach: Dietary modifications (fiber—whole-grain cereals, bran, vegetables, legumes, raw fruit, dried prunes) and bowel training (sit on toilet same time daily for at least 10min, best in AM or PM after a meal)

Nausea and Vomiting (N&V)

ETIOLOGY AND PATHOPHYSIOLOGY

- ■ GI contents ejected through mouth; when ejected with force (**projectile vomiting**); wavelike sensation in throat and epigastrum (**nausea**); complications: dehydration, electrolyte imbalances, and metabolic alkalosis

SIGNS AND SYMPTOMS

- ■ **Common S&S**: Nausea, vomiting, salivation, pallor, diaphoresis, ↑pulse, visible peristaltic waves with projectile vomiting
- ■ **Specific S&S**:
  - ■
  - ■ Curdled vomitus with mucus or vomiting after ingestion of fatty foods (↓gastric emptying or high intestinal obstruction)
  - ■ Vomiting after ingesting food, toxic substance, or drug (allergies, poisoning, drug toxicity)
  - ■ Fever and diarrhea with vomiting (infection)
  - ■ Constipation with vomiting (GI obstruction)
  - ■ Localized abd pain with vomiting (appendicitis, pancreatitis, or peptic ulcer disease)
  - ■ ↓LOC with vomiting (↑intracranial pressure, metabolic disorder)
  - ■ Projectile vomiting (hypertrophic pyloric stenosis, ↑intracranial pressure)

TREATMENT

- ■ Treat cause
- ■ Prevent/treat F&E imbalance (oral rehydration therapy with glucose/electrolyte solution, IV fluids)
- ■ Antiemetic when cause is known (cancer chemotherapy, motion sickness)
- ■ ↑CHO diet to spare protein and prevent ketosis

NURSING

- ■ Prevent aspiration (side-lying with HOB ↑30°); provide physical and emotional support

Assess:
- Pattern and duration of vomiting; amt and character of vomitus
- Vomiting in relation to food, meds, toxic substance
- Presence of constipation or diarrhea
- VS for ↑T and ↑P; I&O; daily weight
- S&S of complications
- Provide hygiene after vomiting
- Reintroduce fluids/foods slowly

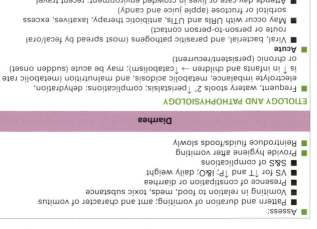

Diarrhea

ETIOLOGY AND PATHOPHYSIOLOGY
- Frequent, watery stools 2° ↑ peristalsis; complications: dehydration, electrolyte imbalance, metabolic acidosis, and malnutrition (metabolic rate is ↑ in infants and children → ↑catabolism); may be acute (sudden onset) or chronic (persistent/recurrent)

Acute
- Viral, bacterial, and parasitic pathogens (most spread by fecal/oral route or person-to-person contact)
- May occur with URIs and UTIs; antibiotic therapy, laxatives, excess sorbitol or fructose (apple juice and candy)
- Attends day care or lives in crowded environment; recent travel

Chronic
- Malabsorption syndromes (fat malabsorption → foul-smelling, bulky stools)
- Food allergies (enzyme deficiency; sugar, protein, or lactose intolerance)
- Inflammatory bowel disease
- AIDS

SIGNS AND SYMPTOMS
- Frequent, watery stools
- >10% weight loss; ↑VS
- Pale, gray, or mottled skin; irritability; lethargy, perianal excoriation

TREATMENT
- Oral rehydration therapy (ORT) with glucose/electrolyte solution, 4–8oz for each diarrheal stool
- Eliminate or restrict cause (antibiotic, laxative, specific food)

NURSING
- Antibiotics only for positive stool culture or if child is acutely ill with fever; avoid ↑CHO fluids (fruit juice, carbonated beverages, gelatin) and caffeinated soda; assess for S&S of dehydration and electrolyte imbalances

- Assess:
  - Pattern and duration of diarrhea; amt and character of stool
  - Diarrhea in relation to fluid, food, meds
  - VS for ↑T, ↑P, ↑R; I&O; daily weight
- Change diaper often and use skin barrier
- ORT and diet as ordered
- Encourage breastfeeding mother to continue breastfeeding
- Teach dietary restriction if ordered

Dehydration

- **Isotonic:** F&E deficits in balanced proportions
- **Hypotonic:** Electrolyte deficit exceeds fluid deficit
- **Hypertonic:** Fluid loss exceeds electrolyte loss; occurs rapidly as total body water in children is 45–75% of total body weight

ETIOLOGY AND PATHOPHYSIOLOGY

- ↓Fluid absorption, ↓fluid intake, GI losses from vomiting, diarrhea, or NGT suction
- ↑Urine output secondary to DM and inappropriate ADH secretion
- Diaphoresis or excessive evaporative losses from fever, hyperventilation, ↑environmental temp, ↑activity, use of radiant warmer or phototherapy
- Hemorrhage

SIGNS AND SYMPTOMS

- Dry mucous membranes, ↓urine output, irritability, lethargy
- S&S vary by degree of dehydration:

Assessment Factor	Mild Dehydration	Moderate Dehydration	Severe Dehydration
% of fluid loss	5–6%	7–9%	>9%
Fluid vol loss	<50mL/kg	50–100mL/kg	≥100mL/kg
Cap refill time	<2sec	2–3sec	>3sec
Skin turgor	↓	Poor	Very poor
Skin color	Pale	Gray	Mottled
Fontanels	Normal or ↓	↓	↓
Eyeballs	Normal or ↓	↓	↓
Blood pressure	Normal	Normal or ↓	↓
Pulse	Normal or ↑	↑	↑ and thready
Respirations	Normal or ↑	↑	↑

TREATMENT
■ Oral replacement therapy (ORT): 50–100mL/kg for mild/moderate dehydration
■ IV fluid replacement for severe dehydration: 1–3 boluses of NS or lactated Ringer's, 20–30mL/kg. Maintenance fluids to ↑extracellular fluid; sodium bicarbonate to correct metabolic acidosis; potassium replacement

NURSING
■ 1g wet diaper weight = 1mL urine; rapid fluid replacement is contraindicated with hypertonic dehydration because of risk of water intoxication; potassium is withheld until kidney function is assessed and circulation improved
■ Administer F&E as ordered
■ Assess:
■ S&S to determine if mild, moderate, or severe
■ VS every 15–30min and then routine; I&O; weight (every 2hr to daily)
■ S&S of excess fluids (**water intoxication**): ↑urine output, irritability, somnolence, headache, vomiting, seizures

Genitourinary Malformations

Estrophy of the Bladder

ETIOLOGY AND PATHOPHYSIOLOGY
■ Absence of portion of abdominal and bladder wall causing eversion of bladder through opening

SIGNS AND SYMPTOMS
■ Presence of defect; leaking of urine, urine smell 2° leaking
■ **Associated defects:** Pubic bone malformation, inguinal hernia, epispadias, undescended testes or short penis in males, cleft clitoris or absent vagina in females

TREATMENT
■ Surgical repair

NURSING

Infant
■ Cover bladder with clear plastic wrap or thin film dressing without adhesive
■ Apply prescribed protective barrier to protect skin from urine
■ Monitor I&O and drainage from bladder or ureteral drainage tubes
■ Monitor bowel function if surgery included resection of intestine
■ Care after surgery for penile lengthening, chordee release, and urethral reconstruction similar to hypospadias repair

Child/Adolescent

- ■ ↑Ventilation of feelings regarding appearance of genitalia, rejection by peers, ability to function sexually & procreate, care for permanent urinary diversion if present
- ■ **Parents**
  - ■ Support parents coping with child with a defect, multistage surgeries, possible need for permanent urinary diversion, impact on child's future sexual functioning
  - ■ Teach care of child, including S&S of infection, clean intermittent catheterization to empty urinary reservoir

Cryptorchidism (Cryptorchism)

ETIOLOGY AND PATHOPHYSIOLOGY

- ■ Failure of 1 or both testes to descend to scrotum; risk for cancer of testes

SIGNS AND SYMPTOMS

- ■ Nonpalpable testes, affected hemiscrotum appears smaller

TREATMENT

- ■ Orchiopexy at 6–24mo to prevent torsion, infertility due to exposure of testes to body heat

NURSING

- ■ Monitor urinary functioning, I&O
- ■ Prevent contamination of operative site by urine and feces
- ■ Apply cool compresses to operative site if ordered
- ■ Administer analgesics and antibiotics as ordered
- ■ Teach parents to assess testes and scrotum monthly and to teach procedure to child when older

Displaced Urethral Openings

ETIOLOGY AND PATHOPHYSIOLOGY

- ■ Abnormal location of urethral opening; may reflect ambiguous genitalia
- ■ **Hypospadias:** Female has opening in vagina; male has opening on lower surface of penis; penis may have downward curvature (**chordee**) 2° fibrous band of tissue; penis appears hooded and crooked; small penis may appear as elongated clitoris
- ■ **Epispadias:** Occurs only in males; opening on dorsal surface of penis; S&S of related defects (estrophy of bladder, undescended testes, short penis)

Urinary Tract Problems

ETIOLOGY AND PATHOPHYSIOLOGY
■ Pathogens (80% *Escherichia coli*) infiltrate structures causing infection and inflammation of urinary tract structures: urethra (**urethritis**), bladder (**cystitis**), or renal pelvis/kidney (**pyelonephritis**)
■ More common in girls 2″ short urethra and proximity of meatus to anus

SIGNS AND SYMPTOMS
■ Symptomatic or asymptomatic; persistent or recurrent
■ Dysuria, urgency, frequency, incontinence, nocturia, strong-smelling cloudy urine
■ ↑Incidence 2–6yr of age

TREATMENT
■ PO or IV antibiotics
■ ↑Fluids (100mL/kg)
■ Extended antibiotic therapy for recurrent infections

NURSING
■ Obtain urine specimen for C&S (catheterization or suprapubic aspiration for child <2yr old) before antibiotic
■ Assess urine for color, clarity, odor, blood, and mucus
■ Encourage fluids
■ Teach: Take complete course of antibiotics; void routinely and on urge, change underpants daily; for sexually active adolescents, teach to void after sexual activity

TREATMENT
■ Circumcision delayed to preserve tissue
■ Surgical repair

NURSING
Child
■ **Postop hypospadias:** Assess for S&S of infection; care for indwelling catheter or stent and irrigate if ordered; avoid tub baths until stent is removed; apply antibacterial ointment to penis daily; administer sedatives, analgesics, and antibiotics as ordered
■ **Postop epispadias:** See estrophy of bladder, p. 88
■ **Parents:** Support coping with child with a defect, multiple surgeries. impact on child's future sexual functioning; teach S&S of infection; care of indwelling catheter (avoid kinks in catheter, never clamp catheter, use urine-collection device in older child to promote mobility); ↑fluid intake; avoid straddle toys, sandboxes, swimming, and contact sports until permitted

Glomerulonephritis	Nephrotic Syndrome
An immune-complex reaction resulting in an exudative process that narrows the capillaries of the glomeruli; is a complication of having an infection in prior 10–14 days. Organism is usually group A β-hemolytic streptococcus	A metabolic, biochemical, or physiochemical disturbance that occurs in glomerular capillary basement membranes. Results in ↑permeability to protein (albumin)
S&S: Periorbital edema in AM, peripheral edema in PM. ↓Urine, dark-colored urine, dysuria. Anorexia, pallor, irritability, lethargy, headache. ↑BP, mild/moderate proteinuria, heart failure. Peak incidence 6–7yr of age	**S&S:** Periorbital edema in AM, generalized edema in PM; → anasarca. ↓Urine output, dark and frothy urine. Pallor, fatigue, irritability, anorexia. Progressive ↑weight, normal or ↓BP, massive proteinuria. Peak incidence 2–7yr of age
Treatment: Symptomatic, recovery usually is uneventful; fluid intake equal to volume of urine excreted plus insensible loss with oliguria. Regular diet, ↓K and ↓Na with oliguria, ↓protein with azotemia. Antibiotic for persistent infection; antihypertensive for ↑BP	**Treatment:** Regular diet, ↓Na diet with anasarca. Corticosteroids, immunosuppressive (Cytaxan) if unresponsive to steroids or for relapses. Occasionally diuretics and/or plasma expanders with anasarca

NURSING

- Monitor VS, particularly ↑BP with glomerulonephritis and signs of infection with nephrotic syndrome; I&O (weigh diapers), daily weight, extent of edema, abdominal girth; urine for amount, frequency, color, clarity, odor, extent of albumin
- Position in semi- to high-Fowler's with ↑R or SOB
- Divide restricted fluid during waking hr; encourage intake of permitted foods; teach fluid and/or dietary restrictions
- Protect edematous skin: Reposition every 2hr, ↑scrotum/legs, clean and dry skin and separate skin folds with cotton clothing
- Encourage rest until proteinuria resolves; provide appropriate age- and activity-level diversions
- Teach parents about meds and their side effects, that irritability and mood swings result from disease and steroids
- Promote a positive body image regarding physical changes related to edema and steroids

Inborn Errors of Metabolism

Galactosemia	Phenylketonuria (PKU):
↑Carbohydrate metabolism due to missing enzyme that converts galactose to glucose. Neonatal screen for galactosemia (Beutler test)	Lack of the enzyme that changes phenylalanine into tyrosine. Neonatal screen for PKU (Guthrie test, McCamon-Robins fluorometric assay test) performed after ingestion of protein
S&S: Variable	**S&S:** Variable
Infant: Vomiting, S&S of dehydration and malnutrition (↓Wt, ↑muscle mass, ↑body fat)	Infant: Failure to thrive, vomiting, irritability, hyperactivity
Even with treatment: Cataracts, ovarian dysfunction, lethargy, growth retardation, motor delay, cognitive impairment	Even with treatment: Blond hair, blue eyes, fair skin susceptible to eczema; red or brown hair in dark-skinned children; bizarre behavior (screaming, head banging, arm biting, disorientation, catatonia); seizures, cognitive impairment
hepatosplenomegaly, jaundice	
Treatment: Eliminate breast milk and foods with milk/ lactose; give soy-protein formula; dietary restriction for life or relaxed as child develops	**Treatment:** ↓Phenylalanine diet (20–30mg/ kg body wt/day) to meet growth needs but prevent mental retardation. Avoid: High-protein foods (meat and dairy). Foods permitted: Most vegetables, fruit, bread, and starches, milk substitutes (Lofenalac). Total or partial breastfeeding OK as breast milk has ↑phenylalanine. Dietary restrictions are lifelong, particularly before and during pregnancy

NURSING

■ Ensure neonatal screening tests are done, particularly for infants born preterm, in the home, or discharged early
■ Identify S&S early as treatment prevents or ↑mental retardation
■ ↑Adherence to drug regimen or dietary restrictions. Use self-monitoring, contracts, and rewards
■ Encourage parents and older child to discuss feelings
■ Refer to dietary counseling and genetic counseling because of genetic transmission; encourage lifelong medical care

92

Upper Gastrointestinal Tract Malformations

Cleft Lip and Cleft Palate
Cleft lip: Unilateral or bilateral fissure in lip; more common in boys
Cleft palate: Unilateral or bilateral, complete or incomplete opening in
soft and/or hard palate; may include lip; more common in girls

ETIOLOGY AND PATHOPHYSIOLOGY
- Congenital malformation caused by genetic aberration or teratogens
(drugs, viruses, or other toxins)

SIGNS AND SYMPTOMS
- Difficulty feeding: ↓Ability to form vacuum with mouth; may be able to
breastfeed
- Mouth breathing with ↑swallowed air → distended abdomen and dry
mucous membranes
- Recurrent otitis media and ↓hearing due to inefficient eustachian tubes
- Impaired speech due to inefficient muscles of soft palate and
nasopharynx, ↓hearing and malaligned teeth

TREATMENT
- Surgical repair
- Possible follow-up with speech therapists and orthodontists

NURSING
- **Preop:**
  - Prevent aspiration: Feed with HOB↑, place nipple (cleft lip/palate nurser,
  Haberman feeder) in back of oral cavity or deposit formula gradually on
  back of tongue via feeding device (Breck feeder or Asepto syringe)
  - Bubble frequently, place in partial side-lying position with ↑HOB, gently
  suction oropharynx prn
- **Postop:**
  - Prevent aspiration (see Preop)
  - Prevent trauma to suture line by limiting crying, if possible, and
  maintaining position of lip-protective device. Use elbow restraints
  if necessary, place on back/side-lying or in infant seat
  - Cleanse suture line after each feeding
  - Assess for ↑swallowing that may indicate bleeding
  - Give analgesic, sedative, antibiotic as ordered
- **Parents:** ↑Ventilation of feelings, show pictures of successful repairs,
teach pre/postop care, encourage cuddling → ↑attachment

Nasopharyngeal and Tracheoesophageal Anomalies

Choanal atresia: Lack of opening between 1 or both nasal passages and nasopharynx

Calasia: Incompetent cardiac sphincter

Esophageal atresia: Failed esophageal development

Tracheoesophageal fistula: Opening between trachea and esophagus

ETIOLOGY AND PATHOPHYSIOLOGY
Congenital malformation caused by genetic aberration or teratogens (drugs, viruses, or other toxins)

SIGNS AND SYMPTOMS
- **3 Cs:** Coughing, Choking, Cyanosis
- **Excessive** salivation and drooling
- **Respiratory** distress
- **During feeding:** Choking, coughing, sneezing, and regurgitation into mouth/nose
- Abdominal distention
- Inability to pass an NGT

TREATMENT
- Surgical repair

NURSING
- **Preop:** NPO, supine and ↑HOB, IV fluids, maintain suction of catheter in esophageal pouch as ordered, monitor I&O and pulse oximetry, suction oropharynx prn, give antibiotics as ordered
- **Postop:** Maintain airway, monitor I&O and daily wt, give gastrostomy feedings until able to tolerate oral feedings, provide mouth care, change position to prevent pneumonia, care for chest tubes if present, give analgesics and antibiotics as ordered, and hold, cuddle, and provide pacifier for nonnutritive sucking
- **Parents:** ↑Ventilation of feelings, support attachment, encourage cuddling, discuss repair, including stay in ICU, teach postop care (suctioning, gastrostomy feedings, skin care)

Hypertrophic Pyloric Stenosis

ETIOLOGY AND PATHOPHYSIOLOGY
- Thickened muscle of pyloric sphincter narrows or obstructs opening between stomach and duodenum; presents 1–10wk after birth

SIGNS AND SYMPTOMS
- Palpable olive-shaped mass just to right of umbilicus
- Visible peristaltic waves across abdomen; colicky pain
- Progressive projectile vomiting; constipation; distention of epigastrum
- Dehydration; ↓wt, failure to thrive
- Metabolic alkalosis (↑pH, ↑bicarbonate, ↓Na, ↓chloride, ↓K)

TREATMENT

■ Surgical repair

NURSING

■ **Preop:** NPO, IV fluids to rehydrate and electrolytes to correct imbalances, NGT to decompress stomach
■ **Postop:** Begin small frequent feedings of glucose, water, or electrolyte solution 4–6hr postop and then formula 24hr later; ↑amount and intervals between feedings gradually
■ **Parents:** Teach care of child, monitor and support child-care skills

Gastrointestinal Problems

Colic

ETIOLOGY AND PATHOPHYSIOLOGY

■ Paroxysmal abdominal cramping; usually occurs first 3mo
■ Multicausation theories: Immature nervous system, cow's milk allergy, ↑fermentation and excessive swallowing of air that ↑flatus, dietary intake of breastfeeding mother, secondhand smoke

SIGNS AND SYMPTOMS

■ Inconsolable, loud crying and pulling legs up to abdomen >3hr per day for >3 days per wk
■ Distended tense abdomen, ↑flatus

TREATMENT

■ Rule out other causes for infant distress; treat symptomatically
■ No evidence-based role for medications

NURSING

■ Obtain a history: determine
  ■ Frequency, duration, and characteristics of crying; relationship of crying to time of day and feedings
  ■ Infant's diet, breastfeeding mother's diet
  ■ Stooling and voiding patterns
  ■ Sleeping pattern, environmental stimuli
  ■ Behaviors of caregivers (methods to ↓crying, response to crying, smoking)
■ Change modifiable causes that may contribute to abdominal pain
■ **Implement 5 "Ss":** **S**waddle tightly in receiving blanket, **S**ucking (pacifier, mother's nipple), **S**ide/**S**tomach lying while monitored, **S**hushing sounds (white noise machine or CD tape), **S**winging (rhythmic movements with bed vibrator, swing, hammock)

- Teach feeding techniques: Proper placement of breast or nipple; feed small, frequent, feeding slowly; burp often; use bottles that minimize air swallowing; maintain calm environment
- Apply pressure to abdomen with hand; massage abdomen
- Eliminate secondhand smoke
- Encourage parent to seek respite from childcare

Obstructions: Volulus and Intussusception

ETIOLOGY AND PATHOPHYSIOLOGY

- **Intussusception:** Proximal segment of bowel telescopes into a distal segment; often at ileocecal valve; presents at 3–12mo; requires nonsurgical hydrostatic reduction or repair
- **Volvulus:** Intestine twists around itself; presents during first 6mo; linked to malrotation of intestine; requires surgical repair

SIGNS AND SYMPTOMS

- Intussusception triad:
- Acute onset of severe paroxysmal abdominal pain
- Palpable sausage-shaped mass
- Current-jelly stools
- Inconsolable crying, kicking, and drawing legs up to abd; grunting respirations due to abdominal distension; vomiting; lethargy; if untreated: necrosis, perforation, peritonitis, sepsis

TREATMENT

- Surgical repair or hydrostatic reduction (intussusception)

NURSING

Preprocedure/surgery:
- NPO; give IV F&E
- Maintain gastric decompression
- Give analgesics and antibiotics as ordered

Postprocedure/surgery:
- Give IV F&E
- Assess VS, amt and characteristics of stool
- Assess passage of contrast material if hydrostatic reduction used for intussusception
- Give oral feedings as ordered; breastfeeding encouraged → ↓constipation
- Encourage parental visits to ↓separation anxiety in older infant

Intestinal Malformations

Imperforate Anus	Megacolon (Hirschsprung's)
Stricture or absence of anus with simple to complex genitourinary and pelvic organ involvement. Surgical repair depends on extent of anomaly	Lack of parasympathetic ganglion cells in portion of bowel leads to bowel enlargement proximal to defect
S&S: Failure to pass meconium stool, abdominal distention, meconium on perineum, in vagina or urine secondary to a fistula	**S&S neonate:** Abdominal distention, vomiting, failure to pass meconium within 48hr of birth, enterocolitis **S&S infant/child:** Occur gradually. Pellet- or ribbon-like, foul-smelling stool; refusal of food; abdominal distention; chronic constipation and S&S of intestinal obstruction
Treatment: Repair with possible temporary colostomy	**Treatment:** Resection with temporary colostomy; stool softeners; dietary modifications

NURSING
- **Preop:**
  - NPO, NGT, IV fluid, and electrolytes
  - Monitor I&O
  - Implement gastric decompression
  - Administer analgesics and antibiotics as ordered
  - Assist with diagnostic tests to identify related anomalies
- **Postop:**
  - Give IV fluids and electrolytes
  - Assess VS, amount and characteristics of stool
  - Extent of surgery dictates care: Anal dilations, care of temporary colostomy, bowel management program; oral feedings as ordered; breastfeeding encouraged because it ↓constipation
- **Parents:** Promote attachment with neonate. Encourage visitation to prevent separation anxiety in older infant

Diabetes Mellitus (DM) in Children

ETIOLOGY AND PATHOPHYSIOLOGY

- Disorder of CHO, protein, and fat metabolism →hyperglycemia that ultimately causes multiorgan complications. For more detail, including information about hyperglycemia, hypoglycemia, DKA, HHNS, Somogyi effect, and dawn phenomenon see Diabetes Mellitus in TAB 6
- **Type 1:** Hereditary and environment; 60% of genetic susceptibility related to human leukocyte antigen (HLA); HLA ↑susceptibility to a trigger (viruses, cow's milk, chemical irritants) that initiates an autoimmune process that destroys beta cells
- **Type 2:** ↓Release of insulin and/or insulin secretion is inhibited or inactivated. Increasing incidence in school-age children and adolescents. More common with obesity, inactivity, ↑fat/calorie diets, and in Native Americans

SIGNS AND SYMPTOMS

- **Type 1:** Onset is rapid and obvious; 3 Ps (polyuria, polyphagia, polydipsia), enuresis, fatigue
- **Type 2:** Fatigue, obesity, recurrent UTIs/vaginal infections; velvety hyperpigmented areas in skin folds (acanthosis nigricans)

TREATMENT

- Dietary/lifestyle changes and medications to maintain normal glucose levels. See Diabetes Mellitus in TAB 6

NURSING

- Design strategies appropriate for developmental and cognitive level, use pictures/play, be interactive
- See DM in TAB 6 and Insulin and Hypoglycemics in TAB 7
- **Preschoolers:** Can be taught about DM and food choices
- **School-age children:** Teach self-monitoring of blood glucose (SMBG), urine testing, and insulin injection (syringe-loaded injector [Injectease] or self-contained device [NovoPen]), S&S of complications
- **Adolescents:** Need for conformity with peers → noncompliance. ↑ Self-care: ↑ motivation with "day off" or occasional dietary treat
- **Self-injection of insulin:** Inject same area for 6–8 injections or up to 1mo; abdomen and thigh best. Use shortest, smallest-gauge needle possible, pinch technique. Insert needle at 90°; track injection sites
- **Nutrition:** Teach glycemic index of foods, appropriate snacks, sugar substitutes with moderation; support personal/cultural preferences
- **Exercise:** Encourage daily exercise; additional food intake $^1/_2$hr before activity and then q45 to 1hr throughout
- **Continued supervision:** Multidisciplinary approach; refer to American Diabetes Association

Congenital Heart Defects

Defects With Increased Pulmonary Blood Flow
VENTRICULAR SEPTAL DEFECT
- Abnormal opening between ventricles; ↑right ventricular pressure results in pulmonary hypertension and right ventricular hypertrophy
- **S&S:** Low harsh murmur throughout systole

ATRIAL SEPTAL DEFECT
- Abnormal opening between atria; right atrial and ventricular enlargement stretches conduction fibers causing dysrhythmias
- **S&S:** Murmur heard high in chest with fixed splitting of 2nd heart sound

PATENT DUCTUS ARTERIOSUS
- Continued patency of fetal connection between aorta and pulmonary artery; ↑left atrial and ventricular workload results in ↑pulmonary vascular congestion
- **S&S:** May be asymptomatic; machinery-type murmur throughout heartbeat in left 2nd or 3rd interspace; bounding pulses; widened pulse pressure

Defects With Decreased Pulmonary Blood Flow
TETRALOGY OF FALLOT
- **4 defects:** Pulmonary valve stenosis, ventricular septal defect, overriding aorta, right ventricular hypertrophy; pathophysiology depends on extent of defects
- **S&S:** Mild to acute cyanosis; murmur; acute episodes of cyanosis and hypoxia (**blue spells**, **tet spells**) when energy demands exceed O_2 supply (e.g., crying, feeding)

TRICUSPID ATRESIA
- Absence of tricuspid valve; no communication from right atrium to right ventricle; incompatible with life without connection between right and left sides of heart (e.g., patent foramen ovale, atrial septal defect, patent ductus arteriosus, ventricular septal defect)
- **S&S:** Cyanosis; tachycardia; dyspnea

Defects With Mixed Blood Flow
- Defects allow saturated and desaturated blood to mix within the heart or great arteries

TRANSPOSITION OF THE GREAT VESSELS

- Aorta exists from right ventricle and pulmonary artery exits from left ventricle; no communication between pulmonary and systemic circulation; incompatible with life without connection between right and left sides of heart (e.g., patent foramen ovale, atrial septal defect, patent ductus arteriosus, ventricular septal defect)
- S&S: Mild to severe cyanosis; heart sounds and other S&S depend on associated defects

TRUNCUS ARTERIOSUS

- Blood from both ventricles enters single great vessel that arises from base of heart directing blood to both pulmonary and systemic circulation; more blood flows to pulmonary arteries because of ↓resistance than systemic circulation resulting in hypoxia
- S&S: Systolic murmur; single semilunar valve produces loud second heart sound that is not split; variable cyanosis; delayed growth; activity intolerance

Obstructive Defects

- Defects cause obstruction of blood flow out of the ventricles.

COARCTATION OF THE AORTA

- Narrowing of aorta near insertion of ductus arteriosus results in ↑pressure proximal to defect and ↓pressure distal to defect
- S&S: ↑BP; bounding radial/carotid pulses; lower extremities have ↑BP, weak or absent femoral pulses, and cool to touch

PULMONIC STENOSIS

- Narrowing of pulmonary valve; resistance to blood flow ← ↑pulmonary blood flow and right ventricular hypertrophy
- S&S: Murmur; mild cyanosis; cardiomegaly or may be asymptomatic

AORTIC STENOSIS

- Narrowing of aortic valve; resistance to blood flow ← ↓cardiac output, left ventricular hypertrophy, ↑pulmonary vascular congestion
- S&S: Murmur; faint pulses; ↓BP; tachycardia; poor feeding; exercise intolerance

Complications of Congenital Heart Defects

HEART FAILURE (HF)

- Heart unable to pump enough blood to meet body's metabolic demands due to ↓myocardial contractility, ↑volume of blood returning to heart (preload), and ↑resistance against blood being ejected from left ventricle (afterload)
- S&S: ↑P; weak peripheral pulses; ↓BP; gallop rhythm; diaphoresis; ↑urinary output; pale, cool extremities; fatigue; restlessness; weakness; anorexia

PULMONARY CONGESTION

- Excessive amt of blood in pulmonary vascular bed; fluid moves into interstitial spaces when pulmonary capillary pressure exceeds plasma osmotic pressure (**pulmonary edema**); associated with left-sided HF
- **S&S**: ↑P; dyspnea; retractions in infants; flaring nares; wheezing; grunting; cyanosis; cough; hoarseness; orthopnea; activity intolerance

SYSTEMIC VENOUS CONGESTION

- ↑Pressure and pooling of blood in venous circulation
- Called **cor pulmonale** when a result of primary lung disease (e.g., cystic fibrosis)
- **S&S**: ↑Wt; peripheral and periorbital edema; hepatomegaly; ascites; distended neck veins in children

Child Nursing Care for Child With Congenital Heart Defects
Child

- Assess for S&S specific to disorder, hypoxia, pulmonary congestion, systemic venous congestion, HF
- Monitor
  - VS, heart and breath sounds, pulse oximetry, ECG
  - Fluid status (I&O, daily wt, maintain fluid restriction if ordered)
  - Electrolytes especially for hypokalemia (↓BP, ↑↓P, irritability, drowsiness) → ↑risk of digoxin toxicity
- Facilitate breathing (↑HOB 30°-45°, avoid constipation and constrictive clothing, O$_2$ if ordered)
- Manage hypercyanotic spells (**tet spell**; interrupt activity, soothe if crying, hold in knee chest position with head↑, which ↓venous return to heart → ↓preload)
- Facilitate feeding (small feedings q2–3h, soft nipple with large hole to ↓work of sucking, bubble frequently, give gavage feedings if ordered)
- Prepare for surgery (age-appropriate teaching)

Parents

- Support grieving
- Discuss specifics of disorder and appropriate care
- ↓Overdependency by child (treat child and siblings equally, age-appropriate goals within child's activity tolerance, consistent discipline) to ↓secondary gains
- Encourage delegation to prevent parental exhaustion

Respiratory Problems

Respiratory Tract Infections (RTIs)

Nasopharyngitis ("common cold"): Inflammation of the nasopharynx

Streptococcal pharyngitis: Group A β-hemolytic streptococcus (GABHS) infects upper airway; can lead to acute rheumatic fever (ARF) or acute glomerulonephritis

Tonsillitis: Inflammation of lymphatic tissue of pharynx, particularly palatine tonsils

Influenza: Influenza virus type A or B causes inflammation of respiratory tract

Otitis media: Acute infection of middle ear usually secondary to *Streptococcus pneumonia* or *Haemophilus influenzae*

Bronchiolitis: Bronchiolar inflammation usually secondary to respiratory syncytial virus (RSV)

Pneumonia: Inflammation of the pulmonary parenchyma

Epiglottitis: Inflammation of the epiglottis

Laryngitis: Inflammation of the larynx

Laryngotracheobronchitis: Inflammation of the larynx, trachea, bronchi. Causative organism identified via C&S; rapid immunofluorescent antibody (IFA) or enzyme-linked immunosorbent assay (ELISA) techniques for RSV detection

FACTORS INFLUENCING OCCURRENCE OF RTIs

■ **Age of child**: <3mo protected by maternal antibodies. Infant and toddler have ↑incidence of viral infections; school-age have ↑incidence of pneumonia and β-hemolytic streptococcus infections

■ **Size of child**: Infants/toddlers have small diameter airways and short, open eustachian tubes ← ↑risk of otitis media

■ **Season**: Viral infections, particularly respiratory syncytial virus in winter/spring, asthmatic bronchitis in winter

■ **Living conditions**: Secondhand smoke, day care centers, multiple siblings, crowded conditions

■ **Preexisting medical condition**: Immune deficiencies, malnutrition, allergies, medical problems (cystic fibrosis, Down syndrome, asthma)

COMMON SIGNS AND SYMPTOMS

■ Irritability, restlessness, anorexia, malaise, chills, irritation of pharynx and nasal passages

■ Nasal discharge, muscular aches, headache, mouth breathing/odor, cough, dyspnea, cervical lymphadenopathy

■ ↑VS; seizures may occur with T >102°F

SPECIFIC SIGNS AND SYMPTOMS

- **Laryngitis:** Hoarseness
- **Tonsillitis:** Tonsils covered with exudates
- **Epiglottitis:** Large cherry-red edematous epiglottis; slow quiet breathing; no spontaneous cough, agitation, drooling, sore throat
- **Otitis media:** Pulling at ears or rolling head side to side, earache, sucking or chewing ↑pain, bulging red ear drum, may exhibit hearing loss, vomiting, and diarrhea
- **Laryngotracheobronchitis (croup):**
  - Stage I: Fear, hoarseness, barking cough, inspiratory stridor
  - Stage II: Dyspnea, retractions, use of accessory muscles
  - Stage III: Restlessness, pallor, diaphoresis, ↑R, S&S of hypoxia and CO_2 retention
  - Stage IV: Cyanosis, cessation of breathing

COMMONALITIES OF TREATMENT

- **Promote respirations:** ↑Humidity with mist tent, humidifier, steam from hot shower in closed bathroom, or saline nasal spray; bronchodilators, ↑HOB, O_2, oropharyngeal suctioning (except with croup syndromes)
- **↓T:** Give antipyretics but avoid aspirin to prevent Reye syndrome. Cool liquids, chest PT to ↑expectoration
- **↑Hydration:** Oral rehydration (Pedialyte, Infalyte), sports drinks (Gatorade, Exceed), ↑calorie liquids. IVF if unable to drink
- **↑Rest:** BR or quiet activity
- **↑Comfort:** Analgesics; heat, cold, gargles, or troches for sore throat. Cough suppressants for dry cough

SPECIFIC TREATMENT

- Judicious use of antibiotics (amoxicillin, 2nd-generation cephalosporin, erythromycin) for bacterial infections; rifampin may be added to eliminate GABHS
- T&A for tonsils and adenoids that obstruct breathing or for recurrent infections
- Antibiotic eardrops, local heat, and myringotomy for otitis media with persistent effusion or hearing loss
- Corticosteroids, endotracheal intubation or tracheostomy for epiglottitis with severe respiratory distress
- Corticosteroids and nebulized epinephrine for croup
- Ribavirin (Virazole) for RSV

NURSING

■ **Acute care:**
■ Droplet precautions
■ Assess risk for obstruction
■ Sputum cultures before beginning antibiotics (best in AM)
■ Support parents/child with frightening SOB or airway obstruction
■ Keep upright (sit on a parent's lap), supine or side-lying position with neck slightly extended (**sniff position**)
■ Humidification and O_2 as ordered; monitor pulse oximetry
■ ↑Fluids to replace loss from fever, perspiration, ↑respirations and to liquefy secretions
■ Manage secretions (nasal aspirator, oropharyngeal suctioning except with croup syndromes); chest PT
■ Antibiotics, decongestants, and analgesics as ordered
■ BR and calm environment; age-appropriate quiet diversional activities
■ **Preventive measures:** Frequent hand washing, containment of soiled tissues, cover nose/mouth when coughing or sneezing, avoid sharing eating utensils, glasses, or towels; formula-feed infants in upright position to ↓fluid entering eustachian tubes
■ **Postop T&A:** Side-lying position with HOB ↑30°; discourage coughing, throat clearing, nose blowing; apply ice collar, ice chips, ice pops, diluted juice (avoid dairy products or red-colored fluids); give ordered analgesics to promote comfort; frequent swallowing may indicate bleeding from operative site
■ **Postop myringotomy:** Place on affected side to ↑ear drainage; apply heat or cold as ordered; clean and apply moisture barrier to protect skin from drainage; recognize S&S of ↓hearing; teach parents to prevent bath and shampoo water from entering ear, feed in upright position, eliminate allergens, and need for follow-up medical care

■ **Asthma**
■ A stimulus → inflammation, which ↑mucus, mucosal edema, and bronchospasm. This traps air in lungs → chronic tissue irritation, scarring, and hyperinflation
■ **Peak expiratory flow rate,** the maximum flow of air forcefully exhaled in 1min, decreases
■ Occurs secondary to allergens (mold, pollen, dust mites, cockroach allergen) or nonimmunological stimuli (infections, exercise, cold air, odors, smoke, stress, dairy products)
■ Characterized by remissions and exacerbations. May be mild and intermittent to severe, persistent and intractable (**status asthmaticus**)

SIGNS AND SYMPTOMS

- Dyspnea, dry cough, prolonged expirations with wheezing, sternal retractions, flaring nares, barrel chest
- **Prodromal S&S of exacerbation:** Rhinorrhea, low-grade T, itching on neck/chest/upper back, anorexia, headache, irritability, restlessness, fatigue, chest tightness, anxiety
- **Progression of exacerbation:** Frothy, clear, gelatinous sputum, productive cough, ↑R, SOB, pale or malar flush with red ears, lips dark red progressing to cyanosis, tripod/orthopneic position, chest hyperresonance on percussion, breath sounds coarse with sonorous crackles
- **Imminent ventilatory failure:** SOB with absence of breath sounds

TREATMENT

Removal of stimulus and medications:

- **Long-term control meds (preventor meds):** Corticosteroids (↓inflammation), cromolyn and nedocromil Na (block mediators of type I allergic reactions)
- **Quick-relief meds (rescue meds):** ↓Exacerbations; β-adrenergics, anticholinergics (↓bronchospasm)
- **Emergency protocol:** 3 treatments with short-acting β-adrenergic spaced at 20–30min, systemic prednisone, and an anticholinergic; hydration with caution to prevent pulmonary edema, O_2 with caution to prevent CO_2 narcosis

NURSING

- Support child and parent in coping with chronic illness and fear related to SOB
- **Prevent exacerbations:** Avoid triggers (dairy, animals); allergy-proof home (eliminate carpets, drapes, down bedding; wet-mop floors). Assess status via peak expiratory flow meter
- **Care during an exacerbation:** Provide a calm presence; monitor cardiopulmonary status; place in ↑Fowler's position; encourage pursed-lip breathing; give ordered meds
- **How to use a peak expiratory flow meter (PEFM):**
  - Measures respiratory volume with 1 breath
  - Begin with indicator at bottom of scale, stand straight, place mouthpiece in mouth, blow out as hard and fast as possible
  - Note result on scale
  - Repeat 3xs, record highest value
    - ◆ Green: Under control
    - ◆ Yellow: Exacerbation and may ↑maintenance dose of meds
    - ◆ Red: Severe airway narrowing and give rescue med

How to use a metered dose inhaler (MDI):

- Delivers premeasured dose of aerosolized med
- Shake inhaler, place canister/spacer mouthpiece in mouth with lips sealed (closed method) or 2–4cm from mouth (open method)
- At end of exhalation, depress canister while inhaling slowly through mouth (3–5sec)
- At height of inhalation, hold breath 5–10sec and then exhale through nose
- Wait 1min between puffs, document results, rinse mouth and equipment after
- Use a spacer particularly with steroids to ↓oral yeast infections
- Take the bronchodilator first to open airway before a corticosteroid

How to use a nebulizer:

- Delivers aerosolized med over several min
- With mask, place over nose and mouth, take slow deep breaths through mouth
- With handheld nebulizer, place between teeth with lips sealed around mouthpiece. Take slow deep breaths; hold inhalation for several seconds, continue until med in chamber is gone

Cystic Fibrosis (CF)

- CF causes ↑viscosity of mucus from exocrine glands and abnormal glandular secretion of ions. It is an autosomal recessive disease.

EFFECTS ON OTHER ORGAN SYSTEMS

- **Respiratory system:**
  - Mucus obstructs respiratory passages ← ↓expectoration, ↓gas exchange
  - Mucus stagnation causes hypercapnea, hypoxia, acidosis, and infection
  - ↑Lung dysfunction → atelectasis, emphysema, cor pulmonale, respiratory failure, death
- **Pancreas:**
  - ↓Secretion of chloride and bicarbonate
  - Mucus blocks enzymes from reaching duodenum ← ↑fat digestion, proteins, and CHO
  - Fibrosis may result in DM
- **Liver:** Local biliary obstruction and fibrosis → biliary cirrhosis
- **Reproductive system:** Delayed puberty; females may be infertile; males usually sterile due to mucus blocking sperm
- **Integumentary system:** ↑Secretion of sodium and chloride in saliva and sweat; hyperthermic conditions → hyponatremic alkalosis, hypochloremia, dehydration

SIGNS AND SYMPTOMS

- Variable; may be asymptomatic for months or years
- Suspected with meconium ileus and failure to regain wt loss at birth, and failure to thrive
- Frequent RTIs, nonproductive cough, wheezing
- Chest x-ray shows atelectasis and emphysema. Pulmonary function tests reveal small airway dysfunction
- Foul-smelling, pale, bulky, watery stools (steatorrhea); stools contain ↑fat and pancreatic enzymes
- Quantitative sweat chloride test (pilocarpine iontophoresis) >60mEq/L
- **Chronic S&S:** ↓Salivation, paroxysmal cough, dyspnea, cyanosis, barrel chest, distended abdomen, thin extremities, clubbing of fingers/toes, rectal prolapse, F&E imbalances, bruising (↓vitamin K)

TREATMENT

- Oral fluids and dornase alfa recombinant (Pulmozyme) to ↓mucus viscosity; chest PT
- Bronchodilators, antiinflammatories and antibiotics
- ↑Protein and ↑calorie diet; salt supplements prn; pancreatic enzymes with meals and snacks to ↓steatorrhea and ↑growth
- Vitamins A, D, E, and K
- Daily aerobic exercise
- Lung transplant

NURSING

- **Child**
  - **Respiratory functioning:**
    - ◆ Assess lung sounds, S&S of respiratory distress
    - ◆ Balance rest/activity; ↑fluids to ↓mucus viscosity
    - ◆ Teach how to ↑expectoration (huffing on expectoration, Flutter mucus clearance device)
  - **GI functioning:**
    - ◆ Monitor wt, abdominal distention, and stools for characteristics and frequency
    - ◆ Monitor for S&S of intestinal obstruction
    - ◆ Teach to ↑protein and ↑calories
    - ◆ Give pancreatic enzymes with food
    - ◆ Ensure adequate salt intake, particularly in hot weather
    - ◆ Use perianal skin barrier to protect skin from GI enzymes
  - **Psychosocial support:**
    - ◆ Provide age-appropriate support to ↑coping with chronic illness, respiratory equipment, invasive procedures, infertility/sterility
    - ◆ Promote a positive self-image

Parents
- Assist parents with shock and guilt (each contributed a gene), chronicity of illness and potential for death
- Teach chest PT (postural drainage, percussion, and vibration); perform daily in AM and PM, between meals to prevent vomiting
- Teach about ThAIRapy vest to provide chest wall oscillation
- Teach diaphragmatic breathing and coughing
- Encourage to support child's independence and limit overindulgence to ↓secondary gains
- Ensure routine immunizations; flu vaccine at 6mo and then yearly
- Refer for genetic counseling and to Cystic Fibrosis Foundation

Blood Disorders

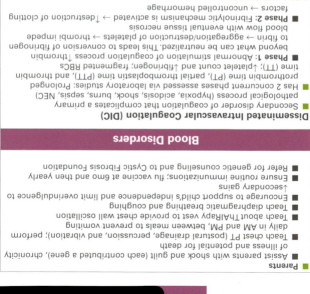

Disseminated Intravascular Coagulation (DIC)
- Secondary disorder of coagulation that complicates a primary pathological process (hypoxia, acidosis, shock, burns, sepsis, NEC)
- Has 2 concurrent phases assessed via laboratory studies: Prolonged prothrombin time (PT), partial thromboplastin time (PTT), and thrombin time (TT); ↓platelet count and ↑fibrinogen; fragmented RBCs
  - Phase 1: Abnormal stimulation of coagulation process ↑thrombin beyond what can be neutralized. This leads to conversion of fibrinogen to fibrin → aggregation/destruction of platelets → thrombi impede blood flow with eventual tissue necrosis
  - Phase 2: Fibrinolytic mechanism is activated → ↓destruction of clotting factors → uncontrolled hemorrhage

SIGNS AND SYMPTOMS
- Petechiae, purpura, bleeding from skin openings (venipuncture, surgical site), ↓BP
- Organ dysfunction related to infarction and ischemia

TREATMENT
- Control of underlying cause
- Platelets, fresh-frozen plasma, exchange transfusions with fresh blood
- IV heparin when not responding to previous therapy

NURSING
- Child: Depends on extent of bleeding, thrombus formation and organs involved; child usually is in ICU; administer IV infusions, blood transfusions, heparin therapy as ordered
- Parents: Support coping with critically ill child

Hemophilia

- X-linked recessive genetic disorder; possible gene mutation
- Males usually are affected and females are carriers
- **Hemophilia A** (classic hemophilia) associated with deficiency of factor VIII
- **Hemophilia B** (Christmas disease) associated with deficiency of factor IX
- Lack of a blood-clotting factor affects coagulation cascade prolonging clot formation and bleeding
- Prenatal testing identifies affected fetus
- Tests distinguish specific factor deficiencies: PT, PTT, thromboplastin generation test (TGT), whole blood clotting time, prothrombin consumption test, fibrinogen level

SIGNS AND SYMPTOMS

- Bleeding from/within body
  - Joints (hemarthrosis) → stiffness, tingling, and ache followed by warmth, redness, swelling, pain, loss of movement
  - Subcutaneous and intramuscular tissue → petechiae
  - Epistaxis
  - Pain
  - Deformities and impaired growth
  - GI tract → black tarry stools, abd pain
  - Brain → headache, slurred speech, ↓LOC

TREATMENT

- Replacement of missing clotting factor
- Analgesics to ↓pain; **RICE protocol: R**est, **I**ce, **C**ompression, **E**levation
- Corticosteroids and nonsteroidal antiinflammatories for hemarthrosis and inflammation of synovial membranes (synovitis)
- Physical therapy; weight control to ↓stress on joints

NURSING

- **Child**
  - Identify bleeding event; provide factor replacement
  - Rest joints; ROM after acute episode
  - Prevent bleeding (noncontact sports, soft toothbrush, water pick, and electric razor)
  - Wear medical alert identification
  - Disclose condition before invasive procedures
  - Support child/adolescent in learning self-care
  - Support coping with chronic disease
  - Explore vocational, financial, and childbearing issues
- **Parents**
  - Encourage ↑ventilation of feelings about child with chronic illness particularly mother because it is X-linked
  - Refer for genetic counseling
  - Safety-proof house and toys, supervise activity
  - Discuss need for multidisciplinary follow-up

Anemia

Iron Deficiency	Sickle Cell Anemia	β-Thalassemia
Inadequate amount of iron to make Hgb, a component of RBCs, which → anemia Caused by ↓dietary iron; infant has iron reserve for only 5–6mo Children receiving only milk have no source of dietary iron (milk babies)	Autosomal recessive disorder: Homozygous patient will develop sickle cell anemia; heterozygous patient will be a carrier More common in African Americans With dehydration, acidosis, ↑T, and hypoxia, HgbS forms long, slender crystals → sickle-shaped RBCs, ↓RBCs, Hgb <9g/dL Cloudy mixture with sickle-turbidity test (Sickledex) for newborn screening Hgb electrophoresis to determine if patient is heterozygous or homozygous **Complications:** → Problems with bones/joints, CNS, spleen, eyes, liver, reproductive system, kidneys, and lungs (chest syndrome: pulmonary infiltrate → chest pain, ↑T, ↑R, cough, wheezing, hypoxia)	Autosomal recessive disorder more common in people of Mediterranean descent ↓Synthesis of β-chain polypeptides → ↓globin molecules Inability to maintain erythropoiesis commensurate with hemolysis, RBC changes, ↓Hct, ↓Hgb, ↑HgbF, ↑HbgA **Thalassemia major (Cooley's anemia):** A homozygous form that results in death without transfusions
S&S: ↑P, pallor, ↓motor development, weakness, dizziness, ↓RBC, ↓Hgb, ↓Hct, ↑total iron-binding capacity, ↓serum-iron concentration	**S&S:** >6mo, failure to thrive, ↑risk of infection **Vaso-occlusive crisis (pain episode):** Sickled cells obstruct blood vessels → occlusion, ischemia, and necrosis. Pain/swelling of hands/feet, abd pain, arthralgia, prolonged penile erection (**priapism**), ↑T **Sequestration crisis:** Pooling of blood → splenomegaly, hepatomegaly, ↓BP, lethargy, hypovolemia, shock	**S&S:** Fatigue, anorexia, ↑T; bronze, freckled skin; splenomegaly, hepatomegaly, thickened cranial bones, malocclusion of jaw, chipmunk-like facies, ↓bone growth, bone pain, delayed sexual maturation

Anemia (Continued)

Iron Deficiency	Sickle Cell Anemia	β-Thalassemia
Treatment: Breast milk or 1L/day of iron-fortified formula for first 12mo. Ferrous sulfate supplements. (May cause → gastric irritation and greenish/black stools) **Nursing:** Give iron-fortified milk/cereals or breast milk. Give iron via a straw to ↓staining teeth. Give with orange juice between meals to ↑absorption. Balance activity and rest	**S&S Aplastic crisis:** Profound anemia due to ↓RBC production and ↑RBC destruction. S&S include lethargy, SOB, altered mental status, and S&S of heart failure **Hemolytic crisis:** ↑RBC destruction → jaundice, reticulocytosis. Suggests coexisting disorders **Treatment to prevent sickling:** O₂, ↑fluids, maintain electrolyte and acid/base balance, hydroxyurea, erythropoietin **Treatment during crisis:** BR to ↓O₂ demands, and rest joints. Give analgesics ↑fluids, correct electrolytes, treat acidosis Blood transfusions or exchange transfusions (replaces sickle cells), antibiotics, O₂ if SOB (O₂ will **not** reverse sickling) Chelation therapy (↓iron overload) **Nursing:** ↓Sickling (prevent hypoxia, dehydration) **During crises:** Give analgesics, oral and IV fluids and electrolytes BR with ↑HOB, support joints on pillows and when moving. Assist with PROM when ordered Give blood transfusions if ordered	**Treatment:** Blood transfusions (may be every 3wk), vitamin C (↑iron excretion), chelation therapy (deferoxamine [Desferal]) Splenectomy if splenomegaly interferes with breathing or if RBC destruction is extreme Bone marrow transplant **Nursing:** Support coping with transfusions and chelation therapy Arrange therapy around lifestyle Support adolescents with potential infertility Teach that screening fetus for β-thalassemia is available

Cancer

Leukemia

ETIOLOGY AND PATHOPHYSIOLOGY

- Unrestricted proliferation of immature WBCs in blood forming tissues
- Leukocyte count is low and immature cells (blasts) are high
- Blast cells compete for and deprive normal cells of nutrients essential for metabolism → anemia from ↓RBCs, infection from ↑neutrophils, and bleeding from ↓platelets
- Leukemic cells may infiltrate other organs (e.g., spleen, liver, lymph nodes, CNS)

CLASSIFICATION

- Acute lymphoid leukemia (ALL) and acute myelogenous leukemia (AML)
- Each have subtypes that have therapeutic and prognostic implications

SIGNS AND SYMPTOMS

- Pallor, fatigue, irritability, ↑↑, anorexia, ↓wt
- Bleeding tendencies (bruising, bleeding from mucous membranes, petechiae, hemorrhage)
- Bone and joint pain; enlarged liver, spleen, lymph nodes
- CNS involvement
- Usually occurs 2–6yr old; onset is insidious to acute

TREATMENT

- Based on staging
- IV and intrathecal chemotherapy given via 4 phase protocol to achieve remission, ↑tumor burden, ↑CNS involvement and preserve remission
- Bone marrow transplant

NURSING CARE FOR A CHILD WITH SCA OR β-THALASSEMIA

- Support parents/child coping with a genetic, chronic illness and potential for death during crises
- Refer for genetic counseling and continued medical care
- Prevent infection (flu and pneumococcal vaccines, avoid sources of infection)
- Balance activity/rest
- Avoid contact sports (prevents splenic rupture)
- Support child and adolescent coping with multiple transfusions, delayed sexual maturation, and body-image issues
- Teach child about disorder and refer to supportive organizations (Cooley's Anemia Foundation)

NURSING

- Depends on side effects of med regimen, extent of myelosuppression, and degree of leukemic infiltration
- Handle gently to ↓pain, bleeding, and fractures
- Emotional support for child/parents coping with dx of cancer, invasive tests, chronic course, potential for relapse and death
- Monitor VS particularly T and BP; provide balance between rest and quiet play
- Teach infection prevention (e.g., hand washing, avoiding crowds and people with an infection)
- Support child coping with side effects of meds (e.g., soft toothbrush, bland foods, small frequent fluid intake, hat to cover hair loss)
- Give chemotherapy and analgesics as ordered

Wilms' Tumor (Nephroblastoma)

ETIOLOGY AND PATHOPHYSIOLOGY

- Malignant tumor of kidney; possible genetic inheritance
- Associated with congenital disorders (e.g., genitourinary problems)
- ↑Mass compresses body tissues, causes secondary metabolic problems
- May remain encapsulated for extended period
- Metastasizes to lung, liver, bone, and/or brain

CLASSIFICATION

- Stages I to V depending on confinement to kidney, extent of metastasis, and if tumor is bilateral

SIGNS AND SYMPTOMS

- Presents as nontender, firm, mass deep within unilateral flank
- Fatigue, ↓wt, malaise, ↑T; hematuria and ↑BP may occur
- S&S of lung metastasis: Dyspnea, cough, SOB, chest pain
- Usually occurs before age 5

TREATMENT

- Radiation or/and chemotherapy before and/or after surgery
- Excision of adrenal gland, affected regional lymph nodes, and adjacent organs
- One kidney excised if unilateral; one kidney excised and partial nephrectomy of less affected kidney if bilateral

NURSING

- Depends on side effects of med regimen and extent of myelosuppression
- Ensure that all health care providers know not to palpate abdomen to prevent dissemination of cancer cells or rupture of tumor capsule
- Emotional support for child/parents coping with dx of cancer, invasive tests, chronic course, potential for relapse and death

Neurological Malformations

Neural Tube Defects

Spina Bifida Occulta and Spina Bifida Cystica

SPINA BIFIDA OCCULTA

Defect of vertebrae with intact spinal cord and meninges

SIGNS AND SYMPTOMS

- May not be visible or may have superficial signs in lumbrosacral area (tufts of hair, angiomatous nevi, dimple, subcutaneous lipomas)
- Progressive disturbance of gait
- ↑Bowel and bladder control

SPINA BIFIDA CYSTICA

- Saclike protrusion on back
- Two most common types:
  - **Meningocele:** The exposed sac contains meninges and spinal fluid
  - **Myelomeningocele (meningomyelocele):** The sac contains the spinal cord, nerve roots, spinal fluid, and meninges. Myelomeningocele is associated with other malformations (intestinal, cardiac, renal, urinary, and orthopedic)

SIGNS AND SYMPTOMS

- Vary; depends on anatomic level and extent of defect; sensory disturbances parallel motor impairments
- Joint deformities are due to denervation to ↓extremities and include flexion/extension contractures, talipes valgus or varus contractures, kyphosis, lumbosacral scoliosis, hip dislocation
- If defect is below 2nd lumbar vertebrae: Flaccid, partial paralysis of legs; varying degrees of ↓sensation; continuous dribbling of urine and overflow incontinence; no bowel control and possible rectal prolapse
- If defect is below 3rd sacral vertebra: No motor impairment; ↓bowel and bladder control

- Monitor VS, particularly T and BP; provide balance between rest and quiet play
- Teach infection prevention (e.g., hand washing, avoiding crowds and people with an infection)
- Teach turning, coughing, deep breathing to prevent respiratory problems because operative site is close to diaphragm
- Support child coping with side effects of meds (e.g., soft toothbrush, bland foods, small frequent fluid intake, hat to cover hair loss)
- Give chemotherapy and analgesics as ordered

TREATMENT FOR A CHILD WITH SPINA BIFIDA OR CYSTICA OCCULTA

- Surgery within 24–72hr decreases stretching of nerve roots and lowers risk for trauma to sac, hydrocephalus, and infection
- Eventually artificial sphincters and reservoirs may be created surgically

NURSING CARE FOR CHILD WITH SPINA BIFIDA CYSTICA OR OCCULTA

- **Infant:** Prevent trauma to sac: keep infant naked in radiant warmer
- **Preop:** Keep infant prone even when feeding
- **Postop:**
  - Place infant in prone or partial side-lying position
  - Use sterile, moist, nonadherent dsg to surgical area to ↓drying; change every 2–4hr
  - Assess for S&S of infection (fever, irritability, lethargy, nuchal rigidity)
  - Assess for leaks, tears, abrasions
  - Keep area free of urine and feces
  - Monitor for hydrocephalus and ↑ICP
  - Use Credé maneuver to empty bladder or straight catheterization if ordered
  - Keep hips in slight abduction; perform PROM to knees, ankles, and feet as ordered; for older child use braces, walking devices, or wheelchair as ordered
- **Child:** Incontinence is most stressful for child's social development; teach clean intermittent catheterization
- **Parents:** Support coping with decision to abort if identified in utero, lifelong care of infant with multiple neurological, genitourinary, and musculoskeletal problems; involve in care; refer to Spina Bifida Association of America

HYDROCEPHALUS

- Abnormal ↑CSF in ventricular system

COMMUNICATING HYDROCEPHALUS

- ↓Absorption of CSF within subarachnoid space
- Often due to infection, trauma, thick arachnoid membrane or meninges

NONCOMMUNICATING HYDROCEPHALUS

- Obstruction of flow of CSF through ventricular system
- Usually due to neoplasm, hematoma, or congenital **Chiari malformation** (herniation of medulla through foramen magnum)

SIGNS AND SYMPTOMS

- ↑Head size in infant is due to open sutures/bulging fontanels
- Sclera visible above iris (**sunset eyes**); retinal papilledema
- Prominent scalp veins and shiny, taut skin
- Head lag after 4–6mo
- May exhibit attention deficit, hyperactivity, mental retardation
- **S&S of ↑intracranial pressure: Infant:** Projectile vomiting unassociated with feeding; altered feeding behaviors; irritability; ↑shrill cry; seizures; **older child:** headache (usually in AM), confusion, apathy, ↑LOC

TREATMENT

- Surgical removal of obstruction
- ↓Excessive CSF by shunting fluid out of the ventricles and to the peritoneum (ventricular peritoneal shunt)
- Shunt revision as the child grows

NURSING

- **Preop:** Maintain in Fowler's position to help drain CSF
- **Pre and postop:**
  - Monitor VS; take serial measures of head circumference (mark site with pen)
  - Assess fontanels for bulging daily
  - Assess for S&S of ↑ICP
  - Support head and neck when holding or moving infant; protect from skin breakdown
  - Keep eyes moist and free from irritation
  - Provide small frequent feedings and schedule care around feedings to ↓vomiting
- **Postop:** Place on unoperative side to ↓pressure on shunt; keep flat to prevent rapid ↓intracranial fluid that may →subdural hematoma
- Monitor for S&S of infection (shunt malfunction, fever, wound or shunt tract inflammation, poor feeding, vomiting, abdominal pain); most common complication 1–2mo after surgery

Anencephaly

Anencephaly is the most severe form of neural tube defect. It is the absence of both cerebral hemispheres with an intact brainstem. The neonate has a small, malformed head and face with a thick neck. The baby is frequently stillborn or may live only several hr to a few days. Death is usually due to respiratory failure.

- **Nursing care** involves providing comfort and support to the infant, parents, and siblings; support the parents as they consider the decision to abort (if condition is identified in utero); to support the parents in coping with realization that their infant has a fatal condition, and to help them consider organ donation.

Cerebral Palsy (CP)

ETIOLOGY AND PATHOPHYSIOLOGY

- Impaired movement, posture, muscle tone, and coordination
- May have intellectual, perceptual, language, and emotional deficits
- Multifactorial causes (e.g., cerebral anoxia most significant; teratogens, brain malformations, intrauterine infections, prematurity, childhood meningitis, toxin exposure)
- Usually diagnosed at end of first year. Nonprogressive. Most children have average intelligence

SIGNS AND SYMPTOMS

- Poor head control and failure to smile by 3mo. Unable to sit by 8mo
- Stiff arms/legs, crossed legs (**scissoring**), floppiness. Pushes away or arches back
- Irritability and crying; persistent primitive reflexes (asymmetric tonic neck, Moro); tongue thrusting and choking after 6mo. Walking on toes; ADHD; seizures
- **Spastic:** Hypertonicity; ↓balance, posture, coordination; ↓fine and gross motor skills
- **Ataxic:** Wide-based gait; poor performance of rapid repetitive movements or use of upper extremities
- **Dyskinetic-athetoid:** Abnormal involuntary movements (**dyskinesia**); slow, writhing movements (**athetosis**)
- Drooling and imperfect articulation (**dysarthria**)
- **Mixed type/dystonic:** Spasticity and athetosis

TREATMENT

- PT (braces, splints); OT (adaptive equipment); speech therapy
- Surgery: Tendon lengthening, selective dorsal rhizotomy
- Meds: Skeletal muscle relaxants, antiseizure, botulinum toxin type A
- Education: Early intervention, individualized education program (IEP)
- ↑Calories for energy expenditure; ↑protein for muscle activity; ↑vitamin B_6 for amino acid metabolism

NURSING

- Teach careful eating (↓aspiration), safe environment, helmet use
- Do not overstimulate; engage in play appropriate for developmental level/ability. Be patient with attempts at speech
- Assist with bowel and bladder training
- ROM to stretch heel cords and prevent contractures
- Teach health maintenance and rehab (PT, OT, speech therapy)
- Teach use and care of orthotics, walking aids, adaptive devices
- Teach about side effects of meds
- Assist parents and child coping with lifelong disability

Cognitive Impairment (Mental Retardation)

- **Mild:** IQ 50–70; educable; mental age 8–12yr; simple reading, writing, math skills. May function in society and have a job
- **Moderate:** IQ 35–55; trainable; mental age 3–7yr; performs ADLs; has social skills. Can work in sheltered workshop
- **Severe:** IQ 20–40; barely trainable; mental age ≤2yr. Requires supportive long-term care
- **Profound:** IQ <25; may attain mental age of ≤1yr; requires total care

ETIOLOGY AND PATHOPHYSIOLOGY

- No characteristic pathology
- Multifactorial causes:
- *Genetic:* Down and fragile X syndromes, PKU
- *Perinatal:* Alcohol/drug use, maternal infections, low folic acid, prematurity, anoxia
- *Medical:* Cranial malformations, meningitis, measles, lead poisoning

SIGNS AND SYMPTOMS

- ↓Functioning in ≥2 areas (communication, self-care, home living, social or interpersonal skills, self-direction, functional academic skills)
- ↑Eye contact, ↓spontaneous activity, nonresponsive to contact
- Delayed developmental milestones; poor results on standardized tests (Bayley Scales of Infant Development 2nd Ed, Wechsler Intelligence Scale for Children-III)
- Passive and dependent to aggressive and impulsive
- Additional problems such as ↓coordination, motor, hearing, and vision
- May have seizures, ADHD, or mood disorder

TREATMENT

- Early identification; early intervention programs
- Individualized education program; PT, OT, and VT
- Placement in day care, respite program, or long-term care facility

NURSING

Child
- Use simple, concrete communication and a variety of senses
- Teach tasks step-by-step while slowly removing assistance (fading)
- Give positive reinforcement for desired behavior (shaping)
- Role-play social behaviors; support independence with ADL; base play on developmental not chronological age
- Encourage peer groups (scouting, Special Olympics)
- Explore sexuality issues with parents and patient (code of conduct, contraception, sterilization, protection from sexual abuse)
- **Parents:** Support parents coping with diagnosis, decision concerning temporary/permanent placement

Chromosome Disorders

TURNER'S SYNDROME

- Abnormal or missing X chromosome; occurs in females

SIGNS AND SYMPTOMS

- **Infants:** Lymphedema of hands and feet; low posterior hairline
- **Children:** Webbed neck; short stature; shield-shaped chest
- **Adolescents/adults:** Undeveloped secondary sex characteristics; amenorrhea; infertile; immature, difficulty with social cues; socially isolated behavior; usually normal intelligence

KLINEFELTER'S SYNDROME

- Extra X chromosome; occurs in males

SIGNS AND SYMPTOMS

- **Infants/children:** no distinct S&S
- **Adolescents/adults:** Tall, thin, with long legs/arms; deficient secondary sex characteristics; infertile; gynecomastia; variable mental impairment; learning disabilities; behavioral problems (↓impulse control, hyperactivity)

TRISOMY 21 (DOWN SYNDROME)

- Extra chromosome 21; occurs in males and females

SIGNS AND SYMPTOMS

- **Infants/children:** Small head with flat occiput; small nose with flat bridge (saddle nose); inner epicanthic folds; small, low-set ears; short, thick neck; protruding tongue; broad, short hands/feet; transverse palmar crease; hypotonic musculature; hyperflexible; variable mental impairment; congenital anomalies, especially heart; ↓immune response; difficulty managing oral secretions; ↑sociability
- **Adolescents/adults:** Delayed/incomplete sexual development; males usually infertile, females may be fertile. Sensory problems (cataracts, ↓hearing); short and overweight

NURSING CARE FOR CHILD WITH A CHROMOSOME DISORDER

- **Child:**
- Maintain airway; protect from infection
- Interact based on developmental level, not chronological age
- Prepare for lack of pubertal changes
- Teach about hormone replacement if ordered
- **Parents:**
  - Provide emotional support; encourage genetic counseling
  - Help set realistic goals for child
  - Support decision regarding placement

Skeletal Malformations

Clubfoot (Talipes Equinovarus) and Developmental Dysplasia of Hip (DDH)

CLUBFOOT (TALIPES EQUINOVARUS)

ETIOLOGY AND PATHOPHYSIOLOGY

- One or more foot is in plantar flexion (downward) and deviated medially (inward); rigid or flexible
- Familial tendency, intrauterine crowding, arrested development

SIGNS AND SYMPTOMS

- Affected foot/feet smaller and shorter with empty heel pad and transverse plantar crease; unilateral affected extremity may be shorter and have calf atrophy; ↑ risk of hip dysplasia

TREATMENT

- Serial casts or surgical correction

DEVELOPMENTAL DYSPLASIA OF HIP (DDH)

ETIOLOGY AND PATHOPHYSIOLOGY

- Abnormal development of 1 or more hip → shallow acetabulum, subluxation, and/or dislocation
- Physiological, mechanical, genetic causes

SIGNS AND SYMPTOMS

- ↑ Abduction of affected leg; audible click when abducting and externally rotating affected hip (**Ortolani's sign**)
- Asymmetry of gluteal, popliteal, and thigh folds; apparent shortening of the femur (**Galeazzi's sign**)
- Pelvis tilts downward on unaffected side when standing on affected extremity (**Trendelenburg's sign**); waddling gait and lordosis when walking

TREATMENT

- Brace, serial casts, surgical correction

NURSING CARE FOR A CHILD WITH CLUBFOOT OR DDH

- Ensure casts are reapplied as child grows; for infant with clubfoot—daily for 2wk and then q1–2wk for a total of 8–12wk; for infant with DDH—hip spica cast changed when needed (3–6mo)
- Ensure that splint (e.g., Pavlik harness) is applied correctly; splint permits some mobility but prevents hip extension and adduction; straps should be checked q1–2wk; worn continuously (3–5mo)
- Perform neurovascular check: Blanching, warm toes, able to move toes, pedal pulse

- **Cast care:** Place diaper under edge of cast; transparent film dsg to form bridge between cast and skin; apply clothing over cast to prevent child from stuffing food or objects down cast; assess for odor
- **Splint care:** Sponge bathe; keep straps dry; place diaper under straps; dress in knee socks and undershirt to prevent skin irritation from straps; inspect skin under straps 3 times/day; massage under straps daily; feed with head elevated; use football hold when breastfeeding; hold and cuddle infant; provide appropriate toys and involve child in age-appropriate activities

Scoliosis

ETIOLOGY AND PATHOPHSYIOLOGY

- Complex spinal deformity in 3 planes: Lateral curvature, spinal rotation →rib asymmetry, & thoracic hypokyphosis
- Multifactorial causes: No apparent cause (**idiopathic scoliosis**), genetic autosomal dominant trait, spinal trauma, concurrent neuromuscular conditions (rheumatoid arthritis, dwarfism)
- X-ray confirms deformity

SIGNS AND SYMPTOMS

- Most seen during preadolescent growth spurt via MD or school-based screening
- Scapular and hip heights are asymmetrical when child is viewed from behind; asymmetry & prominence of rib cage when bending forward
- One breast may be larger; clothes do not fit well (uneven pants legs, crooked skirt hem)

TREATMENT

- Depends on extent, location, & type of curve
- Orthotics (Boston brace, thoracolumbosacral orthosis)
- Spinal fusion for curves greater than 40°
- Exercises to prevent atrophy of spinal and abd muscles

NURSING

- Teach purpose, function, application, and care of appliance
- Check skin for irritation
- Assist with clothing to disguise brace; encourage wearing brace for 16–23hr/day for several yr
- Encourage expression of feelings; role-play how to deal with reaction of others to brace

Postop
- Assess VS, wound, neurovascular status of extremities
- Maintain PCA pump or give analgesics routinely as pain is intense first 48–72hr
- Maintain NGT and urinary catheter and assess bowel sounds and urinary output when removed (↑risk for paralytic ileus & urinary retention)
- If anterior approach used, institute care related to thoracotomy
- Encourage isometric exercises progressing to ambulation & ROM

LEGG-CALVÉ-PERTHES DISEASE

ETIOLOGY AND PATHOPHYSIOLOGY
- Disturbance in circulation to femoral capital epiphysis → ischemic necrosis of femoral head, epiphysis, & acetabulum
- 4–12yr-olds most vulnerable because circulation to femoral epiphysis is mainly by lateral retinacular vessels, which can become obstructed by trauma, inflammation, & coagulation defects; x-ray reveals defect

SIGNS AND SYMPTOMS
- Insidious onset; persistent soreness, ache, and pain in affected hip
- Stiffness, ↓ROM, & limp in affected leg(s)

TREATMENT
- Rest and nonweight-bearing to ↓inflammation
- Containment of femoral head in acetabulum (abduction brace or cast, traction, leather harness sling)
- Surgical repair

NURSING
- Teach use and care of appliance
- Encourage activities adapted to appliance
- Support sense of initiative/industry

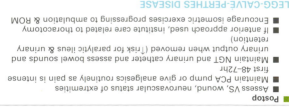

Juvenile Idiopathic Arthritis

ETIOLOGY AND PATHOPHYSIOLOGY
- Infectious agent activates autoimmune inflammation. Familial with female predominance between 1–3 and 8–10yr of age
- Results in chronic inflammation of synovium with joint effusion ultimately leading to erosion, destruction, and fibrosis of articular cartilage, development of adhesions between joint surfaces and ankylosis of joints
- Demonstrates remissions and exacerbations

SIGNS AND SYMPTOMS

- Variable; 1 or more joints involved; joint swelling due to edema, joint effusion, and synovial thickening
- Stiffness (in AM and after inactivity) and loss of motion due to muscle spasms and joint inflammation; weakness and fatigue
- Spindle fingers with thick proximal joint and slender tip
- Joints may be pain-free, tender, or painful
- Diagnosed by S&S and laboratory results (↑erythrocyte sedimentation rate; ↑C-reactive protein; leukocytosis; presence of antinuclear antibodies; positive rheumatoid factor)
- **S&S of systemic arthritis:** ↑T, rash, uveitis, pericarditis, enlarged liver, spleen, lymph nodes

TREATMENT

- Suppress inflammation and pain with nonsteroidal antiinflammatory drugs (NSAIDs; no aspirin to prevent Reye syndrome), slower-acting antirheumatic drugs (SAARDs; e.g., methotrexate, sulfasalazine, hydroxychloroquine, gold); a biological agent that blocks cytokine tumor necrosis factor interrupting inflammation (etanercept), and cytotoxic agents (e.g., cyclophosphamide, azathioprine)
- Corticosteroids used only when other meds are ineffective because of side effects
- PT and OT to ↑muscle strength, mobilize joints, prevent and correct deformities. Splinting of knees, wrists, hands to ↓pain and flexion deformities

NURSING

- Child:
  - Teach to take meds as ordered even during remissions
  - Maintain functional alignment (positioning, splints, firm mattress, periodic prone position, small pillow under head)
  - Apply heat as ordered (10min warm tub bath in AM, warm packs to joints for 20min)
  - Encourage independence in ADLs and exercise program; incorporate play in the program (throwing ball, swimming, or riding bike)
  - Balance activity/rest
  - **During exacerbations:** Give meds to ↓pain, rest joints; maintain functional alignment, encourage isometric not isotonic exercises, maintain contact with school and peers, support developing initiative & industry
- **Parents:** ↑Coping with exacerbations, constant discomfort, risk of overindulgence, seeking alternative therapies

Infections and Infestations

Disorder and Etiology	Signs and Symptoms	Treatment	Specific Nursing Care
SCABIES Infestation due to scabies mite Burrows into and multiplies in epidermis Transmitted by direct contact with infected person, rarely by fomites	Inflammatory response Papules, vesicles, pustules, usually involving, hands, wrists, axillae, genitalia, and inner thighs or feet and ankles of children <2yr Intense itching Mite appears as black dot at end of linear, grayish-brown threadlike burrow	Application of a topical scabicide or ivermectin (Stromectol) tablets Antibiotics for secondary infections	All in contact with infected person must be treated because time between infestation and S&S is 1–2mo Thoroughly massage cream into skin surfaces from head to under feet, keep on 8–14hr, remove by shampooing and bathing Explain that pruritus may take 2–3wk to subside After treatment, all linen and contaminated clothing must be washed and dried at high heat settings
PEDICULOSIS (LICE) Infestation of head, body, or pubic hair by louse Spread by affected personal articles (combs, hats, bedding)	White eggs (nits) attach to base of hair shafts behind ears and at nape of neck Intense pruritus due to crawling insect and insect saliva Papules due to secondary infections	Application of pediculicide (permethrin 1% cream rinse [Nix]) Nit removal with fine-tooth comb	Wear gloves to apply pediculicide Have child's head over sink, back-lying position, eyes covered Remove all visible nits with nit comb Wash all clothing, bedding, towels in hot water and hot dryer; dry-clean unwashables Vacuum rugs, floors, furniture Soak brushes, combs, hats, scarves in pediculicide for 1hr

Infections and Infestations (Continued)

Disorder and Etiology	Signs and Symptoms	Treatment	Specific Nursing Care
BACTERIAL MENINGITIS Acute inflammation of the meninges and cerebral spinal fluid. In neonates may be due to premature rupture of membranes, maternal infection last wk of pregnancy, immune deficiencies In children extension of bacterial infection, neurosurgical procedures, neurological injuries, chronic diseases, immunosuppression	Depends on organism and age Poor feeding, N&V, diarrhea, irritability, drowsiness, headache, respiratory irregularities, positive Brudzinski sign, positive Kernig sign, ↑ICP **Neonate:** ↑Pitched cry, poor sucking, ↓muscle tone, seizures, bulging fontanels **Children:** ↑T, chills, agitation, hallucinations, resists neck flexion or hyperextension, photophobia, cyanosis **S&S specific to organism:** Joint involvement (*N. meningitidis, H. Influenzae*) Petechial/purpuric rash (*N. meningitidis*) Chronic draining ear (*S. pneumoniae*) Spinal fluid culture is diagnostic for organism	Initially broad spectrum antibiotic; specific antibiotic after C&S Dexamethasone to ↓ICP F&E to restore circulating volume while preventing cerebral edema Antiepileptic Acetaminophen with codeine for pain	Prevention: Encourage *H. influenzae* and pneumococcal vaccines Maintain transmission-based precautions for 24–72hr Assess VS, I&O, S&S of ↑ICP, neurological status, Glasgow coma scale, impending seizures or shock Minimize noise, lights, touching Side-lying with slight ↑HOB IV fluids and electrolytes Meds and diet as ordered Support during frightening procedures (lumbar puncture) Support parents as they confront the sudden onset of a serious disease

Infections and Infestations *(Continued)*

Disorder and Etiology	Signs and Symptoms	Treatment	Specific Nursing Care
IMPETIGO: Bacterial infection caused by Staphylococcus or Streptococcus due to organisms from own body (autoinoculations), contact with infected person, superimposed on eczema	Reddish macule becomes vesicular & ruptures leaving superficial, moist erosion; spreads in marginated irregular shapes; lesions dry as honey-colored crusts; pruritus; contagious	Removal of undermined skin, crusts & debris; topical application of bactericidal ointment; systemic antibiotics	Teach parents hand washing & about contact isolation; preventing scratching; administering medications, particularly gently rubbing lesions to remove crusts before topical antibiotic application
CELLULITIS: Inflammation of skin and subcutaneous tissue due to Staphylococcus, Streptococcus, Haemophilus influenzae, enters through break in skin; may be associated with otitis media	Redness, swelling, warmth, and firmness of subcutaneous tissue; lymphatic streaking; local lymphadenopathy; pain; abscess formation	Keep area clean and dry; expose to air and light	Monitor VS & WBC for evidence of systemic involvement; elevate area; apply warm, moist compresses while protecting from thermal injury
INTERTRIGO: Excoriation of body surfaces that rub together; due to excessive heat, moisture and chafing	Red, inflamed, moist, partially denuded skin (intergluteal folds, groin, neck, axilla); obesity and moisture contribute to problem	Keep area clean and dry; expose to air and light	Bathe area daily, pat dry; keep skin folds separated; expose to air and light several times daily for 20min; use superabsorbent disposable diapers and change often

Infections and Infestations *(Continued)*

Disorder and Etiology	Signs and Symptoms	Treatment	Specific Nursing Care
RINGWORM: Fungal infection of the skin *Tinea capitis:* Scalp *Tinea cruris* ("jock itch"). Medical proximal aspect of thigh and crural fold, scrotum in men *Tinea pedis* ("athlete's foot"). Between toes or plantar surface of feet; tinea capitis and cruris transmitted from person-to-person or animal-to-person directly or via contaminated items; tinea pedis often transmitted in locker rooms	Pruritus, characteristic lesions *Tinea capitis:* Patchy, scaly areas of alopecia on scalp; may extend to hairline/neck *Tinea cruris:* Round or oval erythematous scaling patch that spreads peripherally *Tinea pedis:* Maceration and fissuring between toes; pinhead-size vesicles on plantar surface of feet	Oral griseofulvin; local application of antifungal; selenium shampoos for tinea capitis	Teach personal hygiene; avoid pets (particularly cats); not sharing personal items (combs, hats); wearing plastic shoes in swimming areas and locker rooms. Cotton socks and underwear; ↓heat and perspiration; shoes; ventilated and perspiration
CANDIDIASIS (MONILIASIS): Infection of skin or mucous membrane from chiefly *Candida albicans*; grows in moist areas (breast folds, groin, axillae); common form of diaper dermatitis due to wetness and fecal irritants; children with allergies at ↑risk	*Oral lesions:* Painless, discrete, bluish-white pseudomembranous patches on oral/pharyngeal mucosa and tongue *Skin lesions:* Scaly, erythematous skin rash, possibly covered with exudates; painful	Antifungals (oral or topical nystatin preparations); amphotericin B	Teach hand washing and hygiene; Swedish and swallow technique *Diaper dermatitis:* Use superabsorbent disposable diapers and change often; expose skin to air several times a day; apply protective ointment

Integumentary System Problems

Atopic Dermatitis (Eczema)

ETIOLOGY AND PATHOPHYSIOLOGY

- Symmetric cutaneous inflammation with erythema, papules, vesicles, pustules, scales, crusts, or scabs; may be dry or have a weeping discharge; secondary infections common
- Multifactorial causes: Genetics; stress; abnormal function of skin (alterations in perspiration, peripheral vascular function, heat tolerance), environmental factors (dry climate, exacerbations in fall and winter); IgE food sensitization; T-cell dysfunction (allergy to dust, mold, animal hair, chemicals)

SIGNS AND SYMPTOMS

- Characteristic lesions on cheeks, scalp, neck, flexor surface of arms and legs
- Intense itching or burning; facial pallor; bluish discoloration beneath eyes (**allergic shiners**)
- Diagnosis based on history and morphological findings

TREATMENT

- Depends on cause. Topical lotions to hydrate skin, colloid tub baths, phototherapy with ultraviolet light. Avoid precipitating agent
- Meds, including antihistamines, topical steroids, topical or systemic immunosuppressants, interferons, essential fatty acids, topical pimecrolimus (Elide), and systemic antibiotics for skin infections

NURSING

Child

- **Hydrate skin:** Short bath with mild soap (Neutrogena, Dove) and immediately lubricate moist skin (Eucerin, Aquaphor, Cetaphil)
- ↑**Itching and scratching:** Short nails filed to remove edges, cotton socks on hands and pinned to shirt, soft cotton fabrics, and moderate environmental temperatures; teach S&S of secondary infection (honey-colored crusts with erythema)
- **Avoid irritants:** Harsh soap, fabric softeners, bubble baths, excessive bathing, rough/woolen fabrics, double rinse clothing after washing
- **Allergy-proof home:** No rugs, drapes, down pillows, wool blankets; wet dust and vacuum when child is out of house
- **Hypoallergenic diet:** Teach diet; introduce 1 food at a time
- **Parent:** Cuddle irritable child coping with itching; teach that condition is not communicable and scars generally will not occur if secondary infections are prevented

Burns
ESTIMATING EXTENT OF INJURY
- Total body surface area (TBSA) injured represented as a percentage of body surface: Modified rule of nines by %:
  - Head & neck are 18%
  - Anterior trunk is 18%
  - Posterior trunk is 18%
  - Each arm is 9%
  - Each leg is 14%
  - For each year of life after 2, 1% is deducted from head and 0.5% is added to each leg until adult percentages are reached

FLUID REPLACEMENT THERAPY
- Initiated for burns >15–20% TBSA
- Parkland formula often used
- IVF to provide urine output of 1–2mL/kg for child weighing <30kg and 30–50mL/hr in older child
- Urinary output, capillary refill, and sensorium are used to evaluate hydration status and fluid replacement needs

NURSING
- Child
  - Medicate before painful procedures
  - Explain treatments are not punishments
  - Provide age-appropriate support
  - Allow choices whenever possible
  - Encourage expression of feelings. Young children coping with separation anxiety and adolescents developing an identity are most affected
  - Assist coping with physical changes, compression bandages/splints, reactions of peers
  - Accept regression
  - Use behavior modification to motivate
  - Teach age-appropriate fire safety information such as stop, drop and roll if clothing is on fire, not playing with matches, outlets, or stoves
- Parents
  - Support coping with critically ill child, guilt, helplessness, & concerns for child's physical & emotional future
  - Explain multidisciplinary follow-up as scar tissue will require grafts, reconstructive surgery, PT & OT

Poisoning

Chemical	Signs & Symptoms	Treatment	Nursing Care
HYDROCARBONS Kerosene, gasoline, turpentine, furniture polish, cleaning fluids	Coughing, gagging, N&V, lethargy, ↑respiratory rate, cyanosis, substantial retractions, grunting	Gastric lavage; if done, an endotracheal tube is used to prevent aspiration IV fluids O_2	Never induce vomiting to avoid further damage Assess VS and oral mucous membranes for signs of burns
CORROSIVE CHEMICALS Bleach, oven, or drain cleaners, detergents electric dishwasher granules	Severe burning in oral cavity and stomach; white, swollen mucous membranes; edema of lips, tongue, and pharynx Vomiting, hemoptysis, hematemesis Anxiety, agitation	NPO, IV fluids, analgesics O_2 and endotracheal tube prn Repeated dilations or surgery for esophageal stricture	Maintain patient airway, O_2 Give meds as ordered
LEAD (PLUMBISM) Lead in paint, soil, dust, drinking water	Blood concentration >10mg/100mL, anemia and pallor, fatigue, lead line on teeth and long bones, joint pain, headache, proteinuria, lethargy, irritability, hyperactivity, insomnia, seizures	Chelation when blood lead level nears 45μg/dL: succimer (Chemet), British antilewisite (BAL), calcium disodium edentate (CaNa$_2$EDTA)	Screen at 1-2yr old, routinely if ↑risk Eliminate source Ensure adequacy of urinary output before chelation

Poisoning (Continuing)

Chemical	Signs & Symptoms	Treatment	Nursing Care
ACETAMINOPHEN Most common med poisoning in children	History of 150mg/kg for several days, N&V, diaphoresis, ↓urine output, pallor, weakness, bradycardia, liver failure, RUQ pain, coagulation abnormalities, jaundice, confusion, coma	If ingestion occurred within previous hour, activated charcoal may be given If longer, antidote is acetylcysteine Fluids PO or IV	Administer antidote, IVF Assess for S&S of liver failure Teach accurate dose calculation
SALICYLATE (ASA)	**Toxicity:** *Acute:* 300–500mg/kg/day; *chronic:* >100mg/kg/day Diaphoresis, N&V, oliguria, ↑T, hyperpnea, tinnitus, dizziness, delirium **Poisoning:** Confusion, metabolic acidosis, hyperventilation, coma	Gastric lavage, activated charcoal, saline cathartics IVF; vitamin K if bleeding Peritoneal dialysis and hypothermia blanket prn	Assess VS Maintain airway and respirations Give meds and IVF as ordered Care for child when on hypothermia blanket or receiving dialysis

NURSING CARE FOR CHILD WITH POISONING

- **Emergency care**
  - Do not induce vomiting (may redamage mucosa)
  - Identify agent; terminate exposure
  - Prevent aspiration; flush eyes/skin with water if involved
  - Call poison control center (**American Association of Poison Control Centers: 800-222-1222**) and follow their directions
  - Transport for medical care and bring evidence (container, vomitus)
- **Acute care**
  - Maintain airway, monitor VS, assess hepatic and renal function
  - Be calm; do not admonish child or parent
- **Prevention**
  - Teach child not to eat nonfood items (pica) and to follow parents' safety rules
  - Teach parents to keep toxins and drugs in locked cabinet, use child-proof containers

Basic Information

Legal and Ethical Issues

Voluntary admission/commitment: Patient consents to admission; free to leave even against medical advice

Emergency Commitment: Without patient consent when a danger to self/others or is gravely disabled; assessment by 2 mental health professionals; a probable cause hearing must take place within 5 days or less where clear/convincing evidence must be produced to continue in/outpatient treatment

Civil or judicial commitment: Longer than emergency commitment to provide treatment (*parens patriae*: state power to protect or care for pts with disabilities or protect public); procedures vary by state; generally renewable in 90 days/6mo; must follow state rules

Right to least restrictive environment: Restraints or seclusion cannot be used unless ↓restrictive interventions are tried first

Confidentiality: Health Insurance Portability and Accountability Act (HIPAA) of 1996 guarantees privacy/security of health information and enforcement standards; psychotherapy and substance abuse treatment have additional privacy protection

Competency: Patient capable of making decisions about treatment

Informed consent: Right to know risks/benefits to make decisions

Reporting laws: Nurses must report suspected child/elder abuse or neglect, warn a person (and those able to protect person) about a threat made to kill them even if it breaches confidentiality

Nursing Implications

- Know the federal and state regulations/standards regarding legal issues and relationship to information management
- Employ advocacy role
- inform/protect patient's rights (provide information for informed consent, accept right to refuse treatment/meds)
- Maintain confidentiality; consult with agency attorney before releasing information about patient to others or secure signed release from patient
- Enact duty to warn patient's potential intended victims
- Support least restrictive environment, including ↓use of chemical restraints (refer to JCAHO, federal and state standards)
- Know S&S of child/elder abuse (bruises; burns; injuries; inconsistent reporting; signs of sexual abuse; old fractures; exaggerated, absent, hostile emotional response of caregiver; signs of *failure to thrive*)

Mental Health Assessment

Assess the following variables:

Stressors: Assess internal and external stressors

Appearance: Note grooming and hygiene, posture, eye contact, clothing. Is appearance congruent with developmental stage and age?

General attitude: Is patient cooperative or uncooperative, ingratiating, friendly, or distant; hostile, open or defensive, passive, resistive?

Activity/behavior: Congruent with feelings? Note mannerisms, gestures, gait. Is patient restless, agitated, or calm? Is activity hyperactive, aggressive, rigid, or relaxed? Are there tremors, tics?

Sensory/cognitive status: Assess LOC, orientation (to person, place, time), memory (recall, recent, and remote memory), confusion, ability to concentrate

Thought processes: Is thinking rapid, slow, or repetitious? How is the attention span? Assess content: Is the patient delusional, suicidal, obsessive, paranoid, phobic, or expressing religiosity or magical thinking? How is the thinking disorganized? Assess for echolalia, tangentiality, confabulation, loose associations, concrete, clang association, referential thinking, circumstantiality, neologisms

Judgment/insight: Assess decision making, problem solving, and coping ability. Can the patient manage ADL? Does he or she understand the concepts of cause and effect?

Mood: Assess the patient's mood. Terms to describe mood include labile, depressed, sad, happy, anxious, fearful, irritable, euphoric, guilty, despairing, apathetic, angry, shame, proud, relief, contentment, confident, or bizarre

Affect: Affect is the ability to vary emotional expression. Is the patient's affect congruent with mood or is it flat or inappropriate?

Speech: Is the volume and rate congruent with feelings and behavior? Is there pressured speech or aphasia?

Self-concept/self-esteem: Does the patient make negative or positive statements about self? What is the extent of satisfaction with self and/or body image?

Perception: Is there a history of hallucinations, illusions, or depersonalization?

Impulse control: Does the patient exhibit disinhibition, aggression, hyperactivity, hypersexuality, or inappropriate social behavior?

Potential for violence: Risks for violence include depression, suicidal ideation, ↑ muscle tension, pacing, profanity, verbal and/or physical threats

Family/social systems: What is the attainment and maintenance of interpersonal relationships and extent of support system?

Spiritual status: Note the presence or absence of and comfort with beliefs, values, religious affiliation

Defense Mechanisms	
Defense Mechanism	**Example**
Compensation: ↑Capabilities in one area to make up for deficiencies in another	A nonathletic student joins the debate team
Denial: Ego unable to accept painful reality; may assume false cheerfulness	Person fails to seek medical help after weeks of bloody stools
Displacement: Directing anger toward less threatening substitute	Patient throws a telephone after being diagnosed with cancer
Intellectualization: Situation dealt with on a cognitive, not emotional, level	Patient discusses all test results but avoids focusing on fears/feelings
Projection: Attaching to others feelings unacceptable to self	Preoperative patient says to wife, "Don't be scared."
Rationalization: Attempt to logically justify or excuse unacceptable behaviors	Mother of a latchkey 10-year-old says, "He needs to be self-sufficient."
Reaction formation: Inflated reaction opposite to the way one really feels	A person does not like a neighbor but is overly demonstrative and polite
Regression: Retreat to an earlier, more comfortable developmental age	Adolescent has a temper tantrum when the mother says he cannot go out
Repression: Unconscious blocking of unacceptable thoughts from the conscious mind	A woman has no recollection of her father's sexual abuse
Suppression: Conscious blocking of thoughts from the mind	"I'll worry about that after my test tomorrow."
Undoing: Action/words cancel previous action/words to ↓guilt	Husband gives wife a gift after abusing her

Review of Mental Health Disorders

Alzheimer's Disease (Stages)

STAGE 1: MILD
- Patient recognizes a problem
- ↑Short-term memory, mild ↓cognition, confusion, hyperalertness
- Anxiety, depression, invents words that have no common meaning (neologisms)
- Fills in memory gaps with fabricated facts (confabulation)

STAGE 2: MODERATE
- Intellectual decline continues; language disturbance (aphasia)
- ↑Motor activity (apraxia)
- Repetition of same idea in response to different questions (perseveration)
- Failure to recognize words/objects (agnosia)
- Confusion/irritation at end of day (sundowning); sleep disturbances with wandering
- Acting on thoughts/feelings without social control (disinhibition)
- Agitation or aggression, illusions, delusions, and hallucinations

STAGE 3: SEVERE
- Totally dependent
- Complete loss of intellectual functioning
- ↓Bowel/bladder control
- Difficulty swallowing (dysphagia), emaciation
- Immobility leads to pneumonia, UTIs, and pressure ulcers

Signs and Symptoms of Anorexia and Bulimia

Anorexia and Bulimia

	Behavioral	Physical	Psychological
Anorexia	Self-starvation Rituals regarding food, eating, and weight loss Behaviors to ↓weight: purging, exercise, use of laxatives, enemas, and diuretics	Weight loss 15% below ideal Cachexia (sunken eyes, protruding bones, dry skin) Amenorrhea ↓Pulse, ↓body temperature Lanugo on face Constipation Sensitivity to cold	Appears fat to self Intense, irrational fear of being fat Preoccupation with cooking, food, nutrition Delayed psychosexual development Perfectionist, high achiever
Bulimia	Repetitive secret binging and purging Behaviors to ↓weight: purging, exercise, use of laxatives, enemas, and diuretics Fasts to compensate for bingeing	Weight is usually normal; may be ↓or↑ Fluid/electrolyte imbalances (↓K⁺, metabolic alkalosis, dehydration) Menstrual irregularities Dental caries, loss of dental enamel ↓BP, cardiac dysrhythmias Constipation or diarrhea GERD, parotid enlargement	Excessive concern about weight, shape, proportions Lack of control over eating during binging Depression, shame, self-contempt follow bingeing Mood swings, irritability Impulsive, extrovert

Anxiety Disorders

GENERALIZED ANXIETY

■ Excessive anxiety for 6mo, hypervigilance, difficult to control worry, and 3 or more of the following S&S:
  - ■ Restlessness, irritability
  - ■ Easily fatigued
  - ■ ↓Concentration
  - ■ ↑Muscle tension
  - ■ Sleep disturbance
  - ■ Tachycardia, chest tightness
  - ■ Tremors
  - ■ Dizziness
  - ■ Diaphoresis

PANIC

■ Panic attacks lasting from 10 to 30min; see table in Tab 5, p. 139, for S&S

PHOBIAS

■ Unrealistic fear of objects, activities, heights (**acrophobia**), open spaces (**agoraphobia**)

POST-TRAUMATIC STRESS DISORDER (PTSD)

■ Precipitated by a traumatic event
  - ■ Acute: <3mo duration
  - ■ Chronic: >3mo duration
  - ■ Delayed: First evident >6mo duration
  - ■ Flashbacks
  - ■ Anniversary reactions
  - ■ Hypervigilance
  - ■ Nightmares
  - ■ Persistent anxiety

Factor	Mild	Moderate	Severe	Panic
		Levels of Anxiety and Related Signs & Symptoms		
Perception	Broad, alert	Narrowed, focused	Greatly narrowed, selective attention	Distorted, scattered
Motor activity	Slight muscle tension	↑Muscle tension, tremors	Extreme muscle tension, ↑motor activity	Erratic behavior, combative or withdrawn
Communication	Questioning	Pitch changes, voice tremors	Difficulty communicating	Incoherent
Mood	Relaxed, calm	Energized, nervous	Irritable, extremely upset	Panicky, angry, terrified
Physiological responses	Normal VS	Slight ↑ in pulse and respirations	Fight or flight response: ↑VS, dilated pupils, hyperventilation, headache, diaphoresis, nausea, diarrhea, urgency, frequency	Continuation of fight or flight response; may exhibit dyspnea, pallor, hypotension
Learning	Enhanced, uses learning to adapt	Impaired, focuses on 1 issue, selec-tive attention	Greatly diminished, improbable, ↓concentration, ↑distractibility	Impossible, unable to learn

Attention Deficit and Disruptive Behavior Disorders

Disorder	Description
Attention Deficit Hyperactivity Disorder (ADHD)	Before age 7; occurs in at least 2 settings (social, academic, work). **Persistent inattention:** Careless, easily distracted, forgetful, loses things, does not finish tasks, ↓concentration, ↓organization **Hyperactivity:** Runs, climbs, talks, fidgets excessively; impulsive; ↓ability to wait for turn
Oppositional defiant	Pattern of disobedience and/or hostile behavior toward authority figures
Conduct	Pattern of aggressive, destructive behavior with disregard for others and norms of society

Cognitive Disorders

Disorder	Description
Delirium	Acute ↓cognition, lability, fear, delusions, ↑P, ↑R, ↑BP, hallucinations, illusions, disorientation, dilated pupils, diaphoresis, sleep disturbances, tremor. May be reversible (metabolic imbalance, drug withdrawal)
Dementia	Intellectual decline (↓short-term memory, language, insight, judgment), self-preoccupation, may be passive (flat affect, ↓spontaneity) OR irritable (sarcasm, ↓concern for others, paranoia). Progresses from mild to severe; patient ultimately needs total care

Dissociative Disorders

Disorder	Description
Dissociative identity	Persistent/recurrent feelings of detachment from one's body/thoughts
Depersonali-zation	Sudden unexpected travel with ↑ability to recall one's identity/past or assumption of new identity
Dissociative fugue	Memory loss related to an acute, precipitating traumatic event
Dissociative amnesia	Coexistence of 2 or more distinct personalities within 1 person

Factitious Disorders *(Continued)*

Disorder	Description
Malingering	Fabricating a false or exaggerated symptom to gain attention; assumes sick role
Münchausen syndrome	Intentionally causes own illness, sabotages diagnostic tests; **by proxy:** parent creates illness in child and then seeks treatment to gain attention

Grief and Loss

Disorder	Description
Complicated grief	Secondary to multiple losses (traumatic death, loss of partner). Social isolation, substance abuse, morbid focus on deceased, suicidal thought; >3-6mo

Kübler-Ross's Stages of Grieving

Stage and Responses	NSG Implications
Denial: "Not me"; unable to believe loss; may exhibit cheerfulness	Explore own feelings about death and dying; accept but do not strengthen denial; encourage communication
Anger: "Why me?"; questioning; resists loss with hostility/anger	Recognize anger is a form of coping; help other to understand anger; do not abandon or become defensive
Bargaining: "Yes, me, but"; barters for time and may express guilt for past behavior	Assist with ventilation of feelings (guilt, fear, sadness); help with unfinished business if appropriate
Depression: "Yes, me"; realizes full impact; grieves future losses; may talk, withdraw, cry, or feel overwhelmingly lonely	Convey caring (touch, sit quietly); acknowledge sad feelings; accept and support grieving
Acceptance: "OK, me"; accepts loss; may have ↓interest in activities and people; may be quiet or peaceful	Support completion of personal affairs; help family understand and allow patient's withdrawal; support family members' participation in care; do not abandon patient and family

Mood Disorders

Disorder	Signs and Symptoms
Bipolar: Manic and hypomanic episodes	Elevated, irritable mood for 4 days (**hypomanic**) or 1wk (**manic**) alternating with depression plus 3 or more: ↓sleep, grandiosity, flight of ideas, pressured speech, ↑goal-directed activity, distractibility, ↑pleasurable activities with negative results (e.g., buying sprees)
Depressive episodes	Depressed mood for 2wk plus 5 or more: ↑↓wt, ↓↑sleep, psychomotor agitation/retardation, feelings of worthlessness, inappropriate guilt, ↓concentration, suicidal ideation
Major depression	Depressed mood for ≥2wk, ↓pleasure (**anhedonia**) plus 4 or more: ↑↓appetite, ↑↓wt, psychomotor agitation or retardation, altered sleep, ↓concentration, ↓energy, suicidal ideation
Dysthymic	Mild, chronic major depression, lasting ≥2yr
Cyclothymic	Moderate depression to hypomania that may or may not include periods of normal mood, lasting ≥2yr
Postpartum blues	Unstable mood first 14 days after birth, anxiety, fatigue, weepiness, resolves spontaneously
Postpartum depression	Unstable mood 3–12mo after birth. Anxiety, insomnia, ↓energy, ↓concentration, despair about perceived maternal inadequacies
Postpartum psychosis	Rapid onset 2–6wk after birth, insomnia, agitation, hallucinations, bizarre feelings and behavior, risk for harm to infant

Personality Disorders

Cluster A	
Paranoid	Suspicious, fearful, irritable, stubborn, uses projection, hyperalert, aloof, argumentative
Schizoid	Loner, blunted affect, vague thoughts (**poverty of thought**), indifferent to others
Schizotypal	Eccentric behavior, appearance, speech; inappropriate affect; indecisive; withdrawn

Cluster B	
Borderline personality	Unstable relationships, impulsive, intense mood swings, identity disturbance, self-destructive behavior, views things as all good or all bad (**dichotomous thinking**)
Antisocial personality	Manipulates/exploits others without guilt. Lying, stealing, aggressive. Seeks attention and immediate gratification. Does not learn from mistakes
Histrionic personality	Emotional instability, hyperexcitability, attention getting, vain, manipulative, dramatic
Narcissistic personality	Grandiosity, need for attention and admiration, egocentric, arrogant, vain, perfectionist, disturbed relationships, lability of mood

Cluster C	
Avoidant personality	Social discomfort, timidity, loner, fear of embarrassment, hurt by criticism
Dependent personality	Dependent, submissive, indecisive, ↓self-concept, fears rejection
Obsessive-compulsive	Recurrent, intrusive thoughts (**obsessive**); driven, repetitive rituals (**compulsive**); regards self as all-powerful (**omnipotent**) and all-knowing (**omniscient**)
Not otherwise specified	Mixed components of personality disorders: **Depressive:** Dejected mood, ↓self-esteem, negative, feelings of guilt and remorse **Passive-aggressive:** Passively resists responsibilities, envious and resentful of others, sullen, psychomotor agitation/retardation, argumentative, procrastinator

Pervasive Developmental Disorders	
Asperger's	Normal IQ; exceptional talent in 1 area; interpersonal awkwardness; viewed as eccentric; may have bizarre obsessions
Autistic (autism)	Avoids eye contact; dislikes being touched; may whirl/rock/toe walk; slow language development; rigid; tantrums; abnormal speech pattern; repetitive behaviors or words (**perseveration**); may self-mutilate; may be talented (**savant**: math, music)

MENTAL HEALTH

Sexual and Gender Identity Disorders

Sexual disorders	↓Sexual desire: e.g., avoidance of genital contact ↑Sexual arousal: e.g., ↑ability to attain/maintain sexual excitement/erection Orgasmic: e.g., delay/absence of orgasm after excitement, premature ejaculation; female sexual painful intercourse (**dyspareunia**), involuntary perineal muscle contraction with intercourse (**vaginismus**)
Gender Identity	Persistent discomfort with birth gender, desire to change sex characteristics/gender, cross-dressing
Paraphilias	Sexual arousal by: sexual activity with child (**pedo-phila**); genital exposure to stranger (**exhibitionism**); touching nonconsenting person (**frotteurism**); use of object (**fetishism**); watching unsuspecting nakedness/sexual activity (**voyeurism**); inflicting suffering/humiliation (**sadism**), self-humiliation/suffering (**masochism**)

Schizophrenia

■ For 6mo, 2 or more of the positive and negative symptoms

POSITIVE SYMPTOMS: TYPE I

■ Excess/distortion of normal functions; see disorganized thinking and disorganized behavior in Tab 5, p. 145.
■ Delusion: Fixed false belief without external stimulus
■ Hallucination: False sensory perception without external stimulus

NEGATIVE SYMPTOMS: Type II

■ ↓Or loss of normal functions
■ Affective flattening: ↓in range/intensity of emotion
■ Alogia: ↓Fluency/productivity of thoughts/speech
■ Ambivalence: Indecisive because of strong opposite feelings
■ Anhedonia: Inability to experience pleasure
■ Avolition: Unable to initiate/persist in goal-directed behavior

NEUROCOGNITIVE IMPAIRMENTS ASSOCIATED WITH SCHIZOPHRENIA

■ Neurocognitive impairments may occur independent of positive/negative symptoms; however, most are positive symptoms
■ Impairments consist of disorganized thinking and disorganized behavior

Disorganized Thinking

- Concrete thinking: Lack of abstraction
- Circumstantiality: Detailed, long discussion about a topic
- Clang association: Repetition of similar-sounding words
- Echolalia: Parrotlike repetition of another's words
- Flight of ideas: Rapid, repeated change in topics
- Ideas of reference: Neutral stimulus has special meaning
- Loose associations: ↓Connectedness of thoughts and topics
- Neologisms: Made-up words with no common meaning
- Pressured speech: Rapid, forced speech
- Tangentiality: Logical digression from original discussion

Disorganized Behavior

- Agitation: Restlessness with ↑emotions/tension
- Aggression: Hostility with potential for verbal or physical violence
- Psychomotor disturbances:
  - Stereotypy: Repetitive, purposeless activity peculiar to patient
  - Echopraxia: Involuntary imitation of another's gestures
  - Waxy flexibility: Fixed posturing for extended periods
- Regressed behavior: Childlike, immature behavior
- Hypervigilance: Sustained ↑attention to external stimuli

Schizophrenia (Specific Types)

Paranoid: Delusions of persecution, grandiosity, religiosity, or somatization; disorganized thinking/behavior

Disorganized: Childlike affect, socially inept, disorganized speech/behavior, sexually uninhibited

Catatonic: Psychomotor disturbance that may be excessive or involve immobility (**waxy flexibility**), negativism, mutism, posturing, echolalia, echopraxia

Undifferentiated: Delusions/hallucinations, disorganized speech/behavior

Somatoform Disorders	
Body dysmorphic	Preoccupied with real or imagined defect in appearance; hinders work and social functioning
Somatization	Multiple chronic physical symptoms
Conversion	Anxiety unconsciously converted to physical symptoms, rigid, orderly
Hypochondriasis	Abnormal concern about perceived physical symptoms and health despite absence of illness

MENTAL HEALTH

Substance Abuse Disorders

SUBSTANCE ABUSE

- Craving for substance, failure to meet roles, impaired relationships, substance specific S&S, continued use despite consequences (**dependence**)
- Reversible substance-specific syndrome due to recent use (**intoxication**)
- ↑Dose needed for same result (**tolerance**)
- Abuse of 2 or more substances (**polysubstance abuse**)
- Two or more substances produce effect >than sum of each (**potentiation**)
- Substance-specific syndrome due to ↓intake/cessation (**withdrawal**)

ALCOHOL ABUSE

- Excessive, episodic, solitude, and/or morning drinking; slurring; ↑memory; aggressive; blackouts; ↓coordination
- **Korsakoff's psychosis:** Delirium, confabulation, illusions, ↓short/long-term memory, hallucinations
- **Wernicke's encephalopathy:** Neurological abnormalities due to thiamine (oculomotor dysfunction, confusion, ataxia
- **Withdrawal:** Begins in 12hr, peaks in 48–72, improved by 4–5th day; N&V, ↑VS, diaphoresis, anxiety, restlessness, illusions, hallucinations, tremors, GI disturbances, withdrawal delirium (**delirium tremens**) may occur on 2nd but as long as 14th day

OPIATES (HEROIN, CODEINE)

- Euphoria; sedation; constricted pupils; constipation; ↓libido, memory, concentration
- **Withdrawal:** GI cramps, rhinorrhea, watery eyes, dilated pupils, yawning, nausea, diarrhea, diaphoresis

STIMULANTS (AMPHETAMINES, COCAINE)

- Euphoria, initial CNS stimulation then depression, insomnia, ↑appetite, dilated pupils, tremors, paranoia, aggressive
- **Withdrawal:** First psychomotor retardation, then agitation, dysphoria; fatigue and insomnia; cravings; ↑appetite; vivid, unpleasant dreams

OTHER ABUSED SUBSTANCES

- Nicotine; caffeine; hallucinogens (LSD); cannabis (marijuana, hashish); inhalants (glue, lighter fluid)
- CNS depressants (sedatives, anxiolytics); phencyclidine (PCP)

Nursing Care Patients With Mental Problems

General Nursing Care: All Patients

- Maintain safe, supportive, nonjudgmental environment
- Recognize all behavior has meaning
- Encourage ventilation of feelings; do not deny or approve
- Accept/respect patients as individuals; provide choices when able
- Set simple, fair, consistent expectations/limits about behavior; address inappropriate behavior immediately
- Help patient to test new interpersonal skills
- Assist with ADLs as necessary
- Encourage activities that involve patient in recovery
- Teach patient/family about prescribed medications

Nursing Care for Patients With Addictions

- Repeated/chronic use of a substance resulting in dependency
- Associated with substance abuse, antisocial personality
- Use screening tools to assess risk
- Limit noise and light to ↓hallucinations and illusions 2° withdrawal
- Provide and encourage maintenance of a substance-free setting
- Accept hostility without retaliation; set realistic limits to ↓manipulation and/or aggression
- Expect patient to assume responsibility for own behavior
- Encourage patient and family members to attend self-help groups
- Help family members to identify and change enabling behaviors

Assessment of Risk for Alcohol Abuse
CAGE QUESTIONNAIRE

C	Have you ever felt that you should **C**ut down on your drinking?
A	Have people **A**nnoyed you by criticizing your drinking?
G	Have you ever felt **G**uilty about your drinking?
E	Have you ever had a drink in the morning as an **E**ye-opener?

Nursing Care for Aggressive Patients

■ Hostile verbal, symbolic, or physical behavior that intimidates others
■ Associated with substance abuse, conduct disorders, mania, delirium, dementia, paranoid schizophrenia
  ■ Assign to a single room; use nonthreatening body language and calm approach; respect personal space; do not touch
  ■ Provide ongoing surveillance; position self near an escape route; know where colleagues are if help is needed
  ■ Remove potentially violent or violent patient from vicinity of others
  ■ Anticipate needs to ↑stress that may cause anger
  ■ Monitor for frustration, irritation, anger, distorted thinking that may precede violence
  ■ Assist to express anger in acceptable ways (words, writing list of grievances, physical exercise, assertiveness); provide positive reinforcement for acceptable behavior
  ■ Teach to interrupt aggressive patterns (count to 10, remove self)

Nursing Care for Anxious Patients

■ Anxiety ranges from feelings of apprehension to doom. It is a response to a perceived threat to physiological, emotional, or social integrity.
■ Associated with anxiety disorders, phobias, obsessive-compulsive, dissociative, and somatoform disorders
  ■ Assess level of anxiety
  ■ Provide single room, ↓environmental stimuli
  ■ Acknowledge feelings about phobic object or situation
  ■ Recognize somatic complaints but do not call attention to them
  ■ Assist to identify and avoid anxiety-producing situations
  ■ Assist with relaxation techniques to ↓anxiety
  ■ Stay with patient during a panic attack; provide for safety
  ■ Postpone teaching when anxiety reaches severe or panic levels
  ■ Intervene when acting-out impulses may harm self or others

Nursing Care for Patients With Delusions or Hallucinations

- **Delusion:** Fixed false belief without external stimulus (grandiosity, persecution, control, religiosity, erotomanic, somatic, ideas of reference, and thought broadcasting, withdrawal, and insertion)
- **Hallucination:** False sensory perception without external stimulus (auditory, visual, gustatory, olfactory, tactile, kinesthetic, command)
- Associated with schizophrenia, postpartum psychosis, anorexia, depression with psychotic features, drug withdrawal, delirium, and bipolar, obsessive-compulsive, and body dysmorphic disorders
- Recognize and accept that delusions and hallucinations are real/frightening to patient; stay with patient (isolation will ↑hallucinations)
- Identify commands of violence that may harm self or others
- Distract patient from delusions that may precipitate violence
- Point out reality, but do not reason, argue, challenge
- Focus on meaning and feelings rather than content
- Praise reality-based perceptions
- Identify factors that may exacerbate sensory/perceptual disturbances (reflective glare, TV screens, lights)
- Teach self-coping for delusions (recreational and diversionary activities)
- Teach self-coping for hallucinations (exercise, listening to music, "stop, go away!", engage in structured activities)

Nursing Care for Patients With Dementia or ↓Cognition

- Progressive disturbance in memory, speech, insight, judgment, reasoning, orientation, affect and behavior that interferes with ADLs; personality changes (apathy, ↓spontaneity and passivity OR irritability, sarcasm, ↓concern for others, self-preoccupation)
- Associated with vascular dementia and Alzheimer's, Parkinson's, Creutzfeldt-Jakob, and Pick's diseases
- Provide a safe, nonstimulating, familiar environment with consistent routines and caregiver
- Use a calm, unhurried, nondemanding approach
- Consider patient mood and easy distractibility when planning care
- Reorient to time, place, person; use simple language and visual clues
- Promote independence; assist with ADLs
- Encourage reminiscing about earlier years
- Identify events that ↑agitation (environmental stimuli, altered routines, strangers, ↑expectations, "lost" items)
- Involve in simple, repetitive tasks and one-on-one activities
- Promote involvement in therapy (music, pet, current events)
- Support primary caregivers and encourage periodic respite

MENTAL HEALTH

Nursing Care for Patients With an Eating Disorder

- Preoccupation with wt involving ↑ or ↓ intake of food accompanied by wt loss behavior (purging, exercise, abuse of laxatives or diuretics)
- Associated with anorexia, bulimia
- Maintain a matter-of-fact approach, shift focus from food, eating, and exercise to emotional issues
- Assist with contract for behavior-modification program (eating and wt goals with consequences for goal attainment or failure)
- Observe for 1hr after eating to prevent purging
- Provide and encourage intake of nutrient-dense foods
- Support therapeutic interactions (individual, group, family)
- Assist in identifying issues of ↓self-esteem, identity disturbance, family dysfunction
- Provide IV and/or tube feedings as ordered for patient with anorexia

Nursing Care for Hyperactive Patients

- ↑Motor activity and speech, impulsivity, inattention, and expansive and/or irritable mood
- Associated with attention deficit hyperactivity disorder, bipolar disorder manic/hypomanic episode
- Approach in a calm, nonargumentative manner
- Provide a safe, nonstimulating environment
- Channel hyperactivity into safe, controlled activities
- Use easy distractibility to redirect inappropriate behavior
- Keep activities simple, repetitive, and of short duration
- Use rewards (tokens, praise) to ↑appropriate behavior
- Balance energy expenditure and rest
- Provide high-protein/calorie handheld foods

Nursing Care for Patients With Obsessive-Compulsive Disorder

- Uncontrollable desire to dwell on intrusive and inappropriate thoughts (**obsession**); repetitive actions to relieve anxiety connected with an obsession (**compulsion**)
- Associated with obsessive-compulsive disorders, anxiety
- Know patient realizes the ritual is not rational but cannot control it
- Allow performance of ritual until patient develops other defenses
- Limit time and frequency of ritual after other defenses develop
- Intervene when acting-out impulses may harm self or others
- Reduce stress of decision making to ↑anxiety
- Assist to identify and avoid anxiety-producing situations
- Help to identify and use positive anxiety-reducing behaviors

Nursing Care for Patients With Paranoia

- Suspicious thinking that is persecutory (being harassed, poisoned, or judged critically)
- Associated with paranoid personality disorder, paranoid schizophrenia, delusional paranoid disorder
- Respect personal space; do not touch
- Use nonthreatening body language; be calm and reassuring
- Provide environment and activities that do not challenge security
- Recognize and accept that delusions are real and frightening to patient
- Identify presence of dangerous command hallucinations
- Point out reality but do not directly challenge delusions
- Praise reality-based perceptions

Nursing Care for Patients With a Personality Disorder

- Persistent, pervasive, inflexible pattern of inner experience/behavior that deviates markedly from the norm
- Associated with **Cluster A:** (paranoid, schizoid, schizotypal); **Cluster B:** (borderline, antisocial, histrionic, narcissistic); **Cluster C:** (avoidant, dependent, obsessive-compulsive)
- Recognize development of trust will take time
- Assess level of dependence and independence
- Support decision making and independence
- Involve patient in activities that ↑self-esteem
- Engage in social skills training specific to the disorder
- *Cluster A:* See Nursing Care for Patients with Paranoia
- *Cluster B:* See Nursing Care for Hyperactive Patients and Nursing Care for Aggressive Patients
- *Cluster C:* See Nursing Care for Withdrawn Patients and Nursing Care for Patients with Obsessive-Compulsive Disorder

Nursing Care for Suicidal Patients

- Increased risk for suicide is associated with mood disorders; command hallucinations; young adults and adolescents; single older adults (↑men); stress/loss; social isolation; substance abuse; hopelessness or helplessness; serious illness; sexual identity crisis; physical or emotional abuse
- **Levels of Suicidal behavior**
  - **Suicidal ideation:** Thoughts of suicide or self-injurious acts expressed verbally or symbolically
  - **Suicide threat:** Expression of intent to commit suicide without action
  - **Suicide gesture:** Self-directed act that results in minor injury
  - **Suicidal attempt:** Self-directed act that may result in minor or major injury by person who intended to die
  - **Suicide:** Self-inflicted death
- Provide constant observation and safe environment (no sharps); assign to a 2-bedded room
- Identify if patient is giving away possessions or putting affairs in order
- Identify what precipitated or contributed to suicide crisis
- Ask patient if there is a plan and means to carry out suicide
- Encourage patient to write a no-suicide contract
- Focus on patient's strengths rather than weaknesses
- Encourage exploration of consequences if suicide attempt is unsuccessful, impact on others if successful, feelings about death, and reasons for living
- Assist with problem solving; prioritize problems; focus on 1 at a time
- Assist patient to write a list of support system and community resources and how to ask for help
- Ensure family members are aware of need to maintain safety, as most suicides occur within 90 days after hospitalization

Nursing Care for Withdrawn Patients

- Patient retreats from people and reality
- Associated with autism, depression, anxiety, schizophrenia, bipolar disorder depressive episode, avoidant/dependent personality disorders
- Accept feelings of worthlessness as real
- Monitor risk for suicide especially as depression/energy lift
- Sit quietly next to patient, then encourage one-on-one interaction
- Spend time with patient to support worthiness, provide realistic praise
- Accept but do not reward dependence; provide simple choices
- Minimize isolation; involve in simple, repetitive activities
- Assist to identify and replace self-deprecating thoughts with positive thoughts through cognitive restructuring

Therapeutic Modalities

Nurse

- Therapeutic use of self to diagnose and treat human responses to actual or potential mental health problems
- **Nursing:** Health promotion, intake screening and evaluation, case management, support of self-care activities, psychobiological interventions, teaching, counseling, crisis intervention, milieu therapy, psychosocial rehabilitation

Individual Psychotherapy

- Patient and therapist enter into a therapeutic relationship
- **Nursing:** Assist to clarify perceptions, identify feelings, make connections among thoughts, feelings, and events, and ↑insight

Family Therapy

- Family treated as a unit; focuses on dynamics to attain and maintain balance and harmony
- **Nursing:** Help establish boundaries, assess hierarchy/subsystems, ↑communication, ↑interpersonal skills, and promote family cohesion/flexibility (see Group Therapy next page)

Milieu Therapy

- Therapeutic community; social structure is involved in helping process; interactions influence behavioral change
- **Nursing:** Provide clear communication, a safe environment, an activity schedule with therapeutic goals, and a support network

Self-Help Groups

- People have common beliefs, values, and behaviors
- Must desire to change behavior; receive/give assistance to peers; leadership is shared by peers; lifelong process
- **Nursing:** Refer to appropriate group

Behavioral Therapy

- Reward acceptable behaviors so they are reinforced (**operant conditioning**); based on *behavior has consequences;* patients are active participants
- **Nursing:** Establish behavioral contract with goals/consequences; set firm, consistent limits on unacceptable behavior; reward acceptable behavior/achievement of goals (**token economy**)

Group Therapy

- People share thoughts/feelings and help each other examine common issues and concerns

Stages of Group Process

Stage	Characteristics	Nursing
Beginning	Polite and congenial behavior initially; concerned with role and place in group; conflict dominates the end	Provide orientation, set boundaries, help identify purpose and tasks
Working	Develop rules, rituals, behavioral norms; develop cohesive, cooperative relationships; share ideas, experiences, feelings; focus is on the present	Provide structure, model acceptance, facilitate interaction, promote task accomplishment
Termination	Begin to grieve for loss; attempt to reestablish self as individual	Promote summary of group work, resist introduction of new topics, facilitate closure

Psychoeducation

- Educational strategies to ↑information and develop skills (**social skills training**); basis of psychosocial rehabilitation; individual or group
- **Nursing:** Identify readiness to learn, begin at patient level, build on strengths/experiences, individualize plan, give constructive feedback, perform demonstration/return demonstration, role-play; focus on information about etiology, treatment, stress management, prognosis; develop communication, social, and problem-solving skills

Light Therapy (Phototherapy)

- Exposure to bright full-spectrum fluorescent lamps; suppresses melatonin production and normalizes disturbance in circadian rhythms; relieves depression of seasonal affective disorder (SAD); given from 30min to 2–5hr daily; depression begins to lift within 1–4 days; full effect in 2wk; maintained with daily sessions of 30min
- **Nursing:** Ensure ophthalmic consultation for preexisting eye problem; most effective on arising before 8:00 a.m.; sit 3ft from lights; may engage in other activities but must glance at light every few min; monitor for side effects (eye strain, headache, insomnia, irritability)

Electroconvulsive Therapy (ECT)

- A short-acting barbiturate and a muscle relaxant (succinylcholine chloride [Anectine]) given before a brief electrical current is administered unilaterally on nondominant side; current passes through brain to produce a generalized seizure; 2–3 treatments a wk for 3–4wk; alters brain chemistry to improve mood
- **Nursing before ECT:** Witness informed consent; allay concerns and correct myths (memory returns in 6–9mo, not painful); ensure ECG, physical exam, and lab work are done; no food/fluid after midnight; empty bladder; remove jewelry, dental appliances, nail polish
- **Nursing during/after ECT:** Monitor VS before, during, after ECT; insert mouth guard; preoxygenate before and maintain O_2 after ECT; prevent harm during seizure; ensure patent airway after seizure; monitor side effects when patient awakens 10–15min after ETC (headache, muscle aches, confusion, and disorientation; usually disappears within 1hr)

Seclusion and Restraint

- Place in single locked/unlocked safe room (**seclusion**); physical restriction of movement (**restraint**); protects patient/others; standards moving toward "no seclusion or restraint" policies
- **Nursing:** Use less restrictive interventions first; ensure not done for convenience, retaliation, coercion, discipline; when used in an emergency, a licensed independent practitioner must perform face-to-face evaluation (1hr rule); continuous in-person observation of patient for duration of use; when seclusion only is used, audio and video equipment permitted after 1st hour; family must be notified

Occupational Therapy

■ Activities that ↓attention span, ↑motor/social skills, ↑ability with ADLs
■ **Nursing:** Role model, encourage, support, teach, discuss, and promote reality testing of prescribed tasks

Activity Therapy

■ Therapeutic, expressive activity to ↓pathology and ↑mental/emotional health; ↑awareness of feelings, behaviors, thoughts, sensations
■ **Nursing:** Determine level of functioning; provide a variety of groups (recreation, art, music; dance/movement, pet); support efforts; children benefit from play because they are less able to verbalize thoughts/feelings; patients with cognitive impairments do better in less challenging, low-functioning groups

Crisis Intervention

■ Assist to return to previous level of functioning; develop more constructive coping skills
■ **Crisis:** A positive or negative sudden stressful experience perceived as threatening when usual coping does not maintain integrity
■ **Developmental (internal):** Related to life events—adolescence, completing school, marriage, childbirth, menopause/climacteric, retirement, aging
■ **Situational (external):** Related to unexpected situations—relocation, loss of a job, environmental disasters, health problem, bioterrorism
■ **Nursing:** Have patient describe event; support when confronting reality; ↑expression of feelings; clarify fantasies with facts; explore strengths, weaknesses; support systems; assist with problem solving and development of new coping strategies; refer to community resources

Psychopharmacology

■ Drugs that affect emotion, behavior, and cognition; anxiolytics, mood-stabilizers, stimulants, antidepressants, and antipsychotics
■ **Nursing:** See TAB 7—Pharmacology

Renal and Urinary Disorders

Urinary Tract Infections (UTI)

UTIs may lead to bacterial sepsis and kidney failure.

Lower UTI: Urethritis, Cystitis
Pathophysiology
- Ascending pathogens such as *E. coli* cause inflammation of the urethra (urethritis) and inflammation of the bladder (cystitis)

Risk Factors
- Catheterization, female gender, incontinence, ↑age, DM

Signs and Symptoms
- Frequency, urgency, burning
- Bacteria, RBC, and WBC in urine, ↑serum WBC

Treatment
- Urine and blood cultures prn
- Antibiotics, antispasmodics, urinary tract antiseptics, sulfonamides, urinary tract analgesic—phenazopyridine (Pyridium)
- Sepsis requires IV fluid volume replacement, antibiotics, and nutritional support

Nursing
- Monitor S&S, C&S to determine appropriateness of antibiotic, ↑fluids to 3-4L daily, empty bladder q3-4hr, perineal care
- Indwelling catheter: Surgical asepsis during insertion, closed system, secure to leg to prevent movement in and out of urethra, keep collection bag lower than bladder

Upper UTI: Pyelonephritis
Pathophysiology
- Urine reflux from bladder into ureters (ureterovesical reflux) or obstruction causes inflammation of the renal pelvis

Risk Factors
- Calculi, stricture, enlarged prostate, incompetent ureterovesical valve

Signs and Symptoms
- ↑T, chills, N&V
- Tender costovertebral angle (flank pain)

(Continued text on following page)

MEDSURG

Treatment
See Treatment under Lower UTI

Nursing
See Nursing under Lower UTI

Upper UTI: Glomerulonephritis
Pathophysiology
- Infections elsewhere in the body precipitate inflammation of glomerular capillaries

Risk Factors
- Beta hemolytic streptococcal throat infections
- Bacterial, viral, or parasitic infection elsewhere in the body
- Exogenous antigens (e.g., medication)

Signs and Symptoms
- Hematuria, proteinuria, ↓urination

Treatment
See Treatment under Lower UTI

Nursing
See Nursing under Lower UTI

Prostate Disorders

Benign Prostatic Hyperplasia (BPH) and Prostate Cancer
Pathophysiology
Benign Prostatic Hyperplasia (BPH)
- Enlarged prostate → urethral constriction → urinary retention → ↑risk for UTI, hydronephrosis and hydroureter

Prostate Cancer
- Cancerous cells may metastasize to pelvis, bone, lymph nodes, and liver

Risk Factors
- ↑Age, familial history, African American heritage, ↑intake of red meat, smoking

Signs and Symptoms
- Frequency, urgency, ↓stream, hesitancy, nocturia, retention, sexual dysfunction
- **Prostate cancer:** ↑Prostatic specific antigen (PSA)
- **Bony metastasis:** Back/hip pain, ↓weight, fatigue, anemia, ↑alkaline phosphatase

Treatment
- **BPH:** Alpha-blockers (terazosin), antiandrogens (finasteride), heat, lasers or surgery (transurethral resection [TUR], suprapubic prostatectomy)
- **Cancer:** Radical prostatectomy, radiation, and hormonal therapy (orchiectomy and estrogen)

Nursing
- Monitor S&S, indwelling catheter care
- Postoperative Care:
  - Maintain traction on catheter balloon to ↓bleeding
  - Continuous bladder irrigation (CBI) via 3-way Foley to maintain patency
  - Discuss concerns about sexual dysfunction and urine dribbling

Urolithiasis (Kidney Stones, Calculi)

Pathophysiology
- Urinary stasis or chemical environment that → precipitation and crystallization of minerals. Stones form, which obstruct the ureter and result in hydroureter and hydronephrosis
- Components of calculi vary: Calcium with phosphorous or oxalate (75%), uric acid (10%), struvite (15%), or cystine (1%)
- Stones can recur

Risk Factors
- 30-50yr, male gender, dehydration, diet with ↑dairy and vitamin D
- ↑UTIs (struvite), hyperparathyroidism (calcium), gout and myeloprolific disease increase uric acid

Signs and Symptoms
- Pain; depending on stone location, may have little or no pain ranging to severe pain radiating from flank to bladder or genitals
- N&V, hematuria, pallor, diaphoresis, UTI

Treatment
- Opioids, NSAIDs, hydration
- Lithotripsy (extracorporeal shock wave, percutaneous ultrasonic, or laser)
- Calcium stones: ammonium chloride to acidify urine, thiazide diuretics
- Uric acid stones: allopurinol, ↑urine pH
- Diet based on stone composition

Nursing
- Monitor S&S, strain urine, ↑fluids to 3-4L daily
- Control pain
- Calcium stones: Acid ash diet with ↓dairy, protein, and sodium intake
- Uric acid stones: Alkaline ash diet with ↓purine (organ meat) intake
- Oxalate stones: ↓Tea, spinach, nuts, chocolate, and rhubarb intake

Kidney Failure

Etiology and Pathophysiology

Acute Kidney Failure (ARF)	End Stage Renal Disease (ESRD)
↓Glomerular filtration rate due to ↓kidney perfusion, tubular or glomeruli damage, obstruction Moves from anuria (<100mL) or oliguria (<400mL) to diuresis (↑urine output) Progresses to recovery or ESRD	Chronic kidney failure or ESRD due to progressive, irreversible ↓nephron function → uremia, retention of Na, H_2O, K, and P Metabolic acidosis due to inability to excrete ammonia and reabsorb bicarbonate

Risk Factors

Acute Kidney Failure (ARF)	End Stage Renal Disease (ESRD)
Hemorrhage, septic shock, ↓cardiac output, myoglobinuria due to burns or crush injury, nephrotoxic agents, transfusion reaction, calculi, BPH, infections	Diabetes, ↑BP, chronic infections (pyelonephritis and glomerulonephritis), polycystic kidney disease, nephrotoxic agents (aminoglycosides, lead, mercury, NSAIDs)

Signs and Symptoms
- ↓Urine output, ↑BUN, ↑creatinine, ↑K, ↑phosphate, ↓calcium
- Metabolic acidosis: ↓pH, ↓HCO_3, and ↓CO_2; ↑BP, Kussmaul respirations, proteinuria, lethargy, confusion, headache, seizures, nausea, anemia due to ↓erythropoietin, fluid excess (dyspnea, crackles, ↑P, ↑R, distended neck veins)

Treatment
- Erythropoietin; calcium carbonate; antihypertensives
- ↓Fluid, sodium, potassium intake; ↓dietary protein (↓nitrogenous wastes)
- Hemo- or peritoneal dialysis, continuous renal replacement therapy
- ESRD: Renal transplant with immunosuppressives to prevent rejection

Nursing
- Monitor patency of graft/fistula if present (auscultate bruit, palpate thrill; do not take BP in arm with access)
- Monitor S&S and dietary compliance; weigh before and after dialysis
- Complications of hemodialysis: ↓BP, air embolism, dysrhythmias, atherosclerosis, exsanguination
- Complications of peritoneal dialysis: Peritonitis, ↑triglycerides, hernias due to ↑abdominal pressure
- Kidney transplant: Explain need for lifelong immunosuppressive drugs →↑ infection
- S&S of rejection: Oliguria, ↑T, ↑creatinine, flank pain

Fluid, Electrolyte, and Acid-Base Disturbances

Common Imbalances: Fluids and Potassium

Fluid Deficit	Fluid Excess
Hypovolemia: Proportional loss of extracellular fluid (ECF) and electrolytes **Dehydration:** Loss of H_2O only with $\uparrow$Na related to N&V, diarrhea, GI suction, sweating, $\downarrow$fluid intake, diuretics, adrenal insufficiency **S&S:** $\downarrow$Weight, $\downarrow$turgor, dry skin, weak and cramping muscles, thirst, oliguria, postural $\downarrow$BP, $\uparrow$T, $\uparrow$P, $\uparrow$Hct, $\uparrow$BUN, $\uparrow$specific gravity **Nursing:** Monitor S&S, $\uparrow$po fluids, isotonic/hypotonic IV fluids as ordered, prn antiemetics or antidiarrheals	$\uparrow$ECF volume due to heart or renal failure, cirrhosis, $\uparrow$Na, excess IV fluids, $\downarrow$albumin, $\uparrow$aldosterone secretion **Syndrome of inappropriate antidiuretic hormone (SIADH):** $\uparrow$ ADH $\rightarrow$ water retention and $\downarrow$Na due to disorders of CNS and lungs, infections and malignant tumors **S&S:** $\uparrow$T, $\uparrow$P, and $\uparrow$BP; edema, ascites, crackles, jugular vein distention, $\downarrow$HCT, $\downarrow$BUN **Nursing:** Monitor S&S; teach $\downarrow$Na diet, fluid restriction, and Na content of OTC meds; diuretics and potassium supplements if ordered
Hypokalemia	**Hyperkalemia**
Potassium (K^+) <3.5mEq/L; due to vomiting, diarrhea, gastric suction, diuretics, corticosteroids, diabetic ketoacidosis (osmotic diuresis), starvation; hypokalemia $\rightarrow$ $\uparrow$risk of digoxin toxicity **S&S:** Muscle weakness, fatigue, N&V, $\downarrow$GI motility, $\downarrow$reflexes, abdominal distention, dysrhythmias, elevated U wave and flattened T wave on ECG **Nursing:** Assess S&S, teach about foods high in K^+ (melon, apricots, bananas, milk, meat, citrus, grains). Give ordered po/IV K^+ supplements	Potassium (K^+) > 5.0mEq/L; due to kidney disease, burns, crushing injury, metabolic acidosis, adrenal insufficiency, excess K supplements **S&S:** Dysrhythmias; peaked T waves, flattened P waves, and wide QRS complexes on ECG; muscle weakness, flaccid paralysis, intestinal colic, diarrhea **Nursing:** Monitor S&S; avoid salt substitutes and K^+ sparing diuretics with renal disease **Meds:** Calcium gluconate IV, regular insulin with glucose, $NaHCO_3$, exchange resin (Kayexalate)

Common Imbalances: Sodium and Calcium

Hyponatremia	Hypernatremia
Sodium (Na) <135mEq/L	Sodium (Na) >145mEq/L
Secondary to vomiting, diarrhea, gastric suction, sweating, excess intake of Na-free fluids, diuretics, renal disease, adrenal insufficiency, SIADH	Water loss secondary to diarrhea, ↑fluid intake, heat stroke, excess Na intake (secondary to near drowning in ocean, Na bicarbonate, hypertonic NaCl)
S&S: Muscle cramps, weakness, confusion, seizures, ↑ICP (papilledema, headache, confusion, seizures)	**S&S:** Thirst, ↑T, ↑P, ↑BP, dry, sticky mucous membranes; ↑reflexes, restlessness, ↑reflexes, seizures
Nursing: ↑Na intake, give IVF (NS) as ordered, ↑fluids to 800mL/daily	**Nursing:** Monitor S&S; give IVF (D₅W or hypotonic solution) and diuretics as ordered

Hypocalcemia	Hypercalcemia
Calcium (Ca) <8.5mEq/dL	Calcium (Ca) <10.5mEq/dL
Related to hypoparathyroidism, renal failure, malabsorption, ↓albumin, ↑vitamin D, alkalosis, pancreatitis, meds (furosemide, steroids, cisplatin, mithramycin, INH)	Related to immobility, malignant tumors, hyperparathyroidism, meds (thiazide diuretics, lithium, excess calcium or vitamin D supplements)
S&S: Paresthesias, tetany, facial nerve twitching (**Chvostek's sign**), carpopedal spasm (**Trousseau's sign**), ↑ST segment on ECG, confusion, seizures	**S&S:** Deep bone pain, flank pain (due to renal calculi), constipation, vomiting, ↓reflexes, ↑urine calcium (**Sulkowitch test**) ↑hyperparathyroid hormone (PTH) levels; ↑PTH levels (with malignancy); osteoporosis
Nursing: Monitor S&S; give calcium supplements and vitamin D as ordered; teach high-calcium foods (milk, salmon, green leafy vegetables, sardines)	**Nursing:** Monitor S&S; ↑fluids; ↑fiber; give ordered IVF and meds (mithramycin, calcitonin, furosemide, biphosphonate)

Common Imbalances: Acid-Base

Metabolic Acidosis	Metabolic Alkalosis
Serum pH <7.35 and HCO_3 <22mEq/L; related to ↑acid (ASA poisoning, lactic or ketoacidosis, uremia); ↓HCO_3 (diarrhea, chlorides, diuretics); hypoproteinemia **S&S:** Headache; confusion; fruity breath; ↑rate and ↑depth of respirations (**Kussmaul respirations**) → ↓CO_2, ↓K^+ (shifts into cell) → N&V and dysrhythmias **Nursing:** Monitor S&S and K^+ levels, give $NaHCO_3$ if ordered, supportive care for underlying problem	Serum pH >7.45 and HCO_3 >26mEq/L; secondary to loss of acidic gastric secretions (vomiting or suction), thiazide and loop diuretics (↓serum K^+ causes K^+ to leave cells and H^+ to enter), ↑intake of sodium bicarbonate **S&S:** Paresthesias, tremors, shallow respirations → ↑CO_2, dizziness, confusion, ↓GI motility, ↓K^+ **Nursing:** Monitor S&S; give NaCl fluids, KCl replacement, and H_2 antagonists (↓acid loss from GI suction) as ordered

Respiratory Acidosis	Respiratory Alkalosis
Serum pH <7.35 and $PaCO_2$ >42mmHg; ↓ventilation and CO_2 retention from pulmonary edema, pneumonia, ARDS, narcotic overdose, aspiration, emphysema, obstructed airway, neuromuscular disease, apnea **S&S:** SOB; ↑P, ↑R, ↑BP; restlessness; disorientation; ↑K^+; signs of ↑ICP (secondary to cerebral edema) **Nursing:** Monitor S&S, care for underlying cause (antibiotics, thrombolytics, bronchodilators), ↑oxygenation (suction airway, Fowler's position, mechanical ventilation)	Serum pH >7.45 and $PaCO_2$ <38mmHg; caused by hyperventilation (from anxiety), hypoxemia, excess mechanical ventilation **S&S:** ↑P, ↓K^+, ↓Ca, paresthesias, lightheadedness, dysrhythmias, ↓LOC **Nursing:** Monitor S&S, teach to breathe slowly or breathe in paper bag, give sedative as ordered, mechanical ventilator settings may have to ↓rate and/or depth

Integumentary Disorders

Burns

Thermal, electrical, or chemical trauma → tissue destruction; intensity and duration of heat determine depth of destruction; prognosis depends on location and % of total body surface area (TBSA) involved.

Terms

Extent of burn (rule of nines): Body divided into sections by % to quickly assess TBSA involved: head and neck (9%), each arm (9%), anterior trunk (18%), posterior trunk (18%), each leg (18%), perineum (1%)

- **Minor:** <15% TBSA: face, hands, feet, and genitals not involved
- **Moderate:** Partial thickness 15-25% or full thickness <10%
- **Major:** Partial thickness >25%; full thickness >10%; burns of face, hands, feet, or genitals, other complications

Depth of burn:

- **Partial-thickness (superficial):** Includes epidermis, may include top layer of dermis; erythema, pain, blanching with pressure
- **Partial-thickness (deep):** Includes deeper layer of dermis; erythema, hypersensitive to touch/air, moderate to severe pain, moist blebs, blisters
- **Full-thickness:** Extends through dermis and may involve underlying tissue; pale, white, or brown charred appearance (eschar), edema, absence of pain but severe pain in surrounding tissue, burn odor
- **Inhalation injury:** Facial burns, singed nostril hair, sooty sputum, voice change, blisters in mouth or throat, dyspnea

Burn Phases

Emergent or Immediate Resuscitative Phase
Onset of injury to 5 or more days; usually 24-48hr; from fluid loss and edema formation until diuresis begins

Acute Phase
Weeks or months; from mobilization of extracellular fluid to diuresis; burned area is covered by skin grafts or until wounds heal

Rehabilitation Phase
Two wk to 2-3mo; major wound closure to achievement of maximal physical and psychosocial adjustment; mature healing of skin may take 6mo-2yr

Signs and Symptoms

Emergent or immediate resuscitative phase: Shock from pain and hypovolemia; fluid shift to interstitial and 3rd spaces; edema; adynamic ileus; shivering related to heat loss, anxiety, pain; altered mental state (hypoxia due to smoke inhalation, pain meds); ↑Hct; impairment of immune system (↑WBC)

- **Acute phase:** ↓Edema; necrotic tissue sloughs; granulation occurs in partial-thickness burns (10-14 days)
- **Rehabilitation phase:** Flat, pink new skin becomes raised and hyperemic in 4-6wk and will cause joint flexion and fixation (**contracture**) if not prevented; altered contour (slightly elevated and enlarged over burn injury) minimized with pressure; pain replaced by itchiness

Treatment

- **At the scene of burn:** Put out flames; maintain airway, breathing, circulation; first aid to prevent shock and respiratory distress; apply cool water briefly to ↓trauma and pain (avoid ice → ↑damage); remove clothing and jewelry to prevent constriction related to edema; leave adherent clothing; cover with sterile/clean dressing (no ointments); rapid sustained flushing of skin/eyes if chemical burn
- **In the hospital:** May require intubation, O_2, mechanical ventilator; extent and depth of burns assessed; hemodynamic monitoring; fluid replaced using an established formula ($1/2$ of fluids in first 8hr and other $1/2$ over next 16hr); prevention of electrolyte imbalance (hyper/hypokalemia and hyper/hyponatremia); IV narcotic analgesics; wound care; tetanus toxoid; ECG for electrical burns; meds to prevent Curling's ulcer; ↑calorie, ↑protein diet, vitamins and iron; pressure garments (↓scars); splints (↓contractures)
- **During rehabilitation:** PT, OT, vocational education; reconstruction (cosmetic, functional); counseling to manage ↓function, disfigurement, economic burden, and return to work

Nursing Care

- **Emergent or immediate resuscitative phase:** Maintain respirations; maintain patent airway (suction, endotracheal tube, mechanical ventilator); monitor ABGs, O_2 sat, breath sounds; place in Fowler's position; ↑coughing; teach incentive spirometry; monitor fluid shift from intravascular to interstitial space
- **Acute phase:** Monitor fluid shift from interstitial to intravascular space
- **All Phases**
  - **Maintain fluid balance:** Monitor S&S of fluid shifts, edema, daily weight, I&O, hemodynamic status; give po fluids when ordered
  - **Maintain circulation:** Provide IV F&E, colloids as ordered, maintain urinary output ≥30-50mL/hr, systolic BP ≥100mmHg, and pulse ≤120bpm
  - **Prevent infection:** Assess for S&S of infection (↑T and ↑WBC, wound bed and donor sites for purulent drainage, edema, redness); use contact precautions; give systemic/topical antimicrobials/antibiotics; provide surgical aseptic wound care as ordered
  - **Manage pain:** Give pain meds before procedures and routinely before pain↑; use nonpharmacological interventions (distraction); use lifting sheet; keep room temperature 80-85°F, humidity >40%, prevent drafts

(Continued text on following page)

Hormonal Disorders

Addison's Disease

Etiology and Pathophysiology

- An adrenocortical disorder exhibited by ↓secretion of adrenocortical hormones — ↓glucocorticoids, mineralocorticoids (aldosterone), and androgens, which ← ↑stress response
- Occurs secondary to surgical removal of adrenal glands, autoimmune or idiopathic causes, abrupt cessation of steroid therapy, or infection

Signs and Symptoms

- ↑K+, ↑Na, dehydration,↓serum glucose, weakness, diarrhea, confusion
- ↓BP,↑weight, bronze-colored skin
- ↑ACTH, ↓serum cortisol, ↓17-ketosteroids, ↓17-hydroxysteroids
- **Addisonian crisis:** Pallor or cyanosis, anxiety, ↑P, ↑R, ↓BP secondary to acute stress (surgery, emotions, cold exposure, infection)

Treatment

- Glucocorticoid and mineralocorticoid replacement (↑dose under stress to ↑risk of Addisonian crisis)
- F&E replacement

Nursing

- Monitor for S&S of Addisonian crisis
- Encourage ↑protein and ↑carbohydrate diet with added salt
- Schedule rest periods
- Teach need for lifelong therapy, avoidance of stress, and use of medical alert band

---

- **Maintain nutrition:** NPO initially, high-calorie, high-protein diet with supplements when able, tube feedings or parenteral nutrition
- **Provide emotional support:** Address fear, grief, altered role, body image (explain that edema will subside in 2-4 days); explain all care
- **Maintain bowel function:** Assess bowel function, maintain NGT to decompression (↓N&V, aspiration, ileus formation)
- **Ongoing care:** Assist with hydrotherapy, debridement, grafting; plan for rest; maintain mobility and prevent contractures (positioning, splints, ambulation, ROM); teach use of pressure garments and skin lubrication; ↑self-care activities when able
- **Rehabilitation phase:** Continue monitoring for infection and providing nutritional support until skin coverage is achieved; protect new skin from injury; teach: self-care, wound care; reassure appearance will continue to improve over time; refer to support group.

Cushing's Syndrome

Etiology and Pathophysiology
- An adrenocortical disorder exhibited by ↑secretion of cortical hormones (androgens, mineralocorticoids, glucocorticoids) → ↓immune response, ↑Na, water retention, ↑serum glucose
- Occurs secondary to adrenal tumor, or ↑ACTH from pituitary, steroid therapy
- ↑Risk women 20-40yr

Signs and Symptoms
- ↓K⁺, ↑Na, hypervolemia, edema
- Truncal obesity, buffalo hump, moon face, acne, hirsutism, purple abdominal striae
- ↓Libido
- Muscle wasting → thin extremities
- ↑Glucose, ↑serum cortisol, ↑17-ketosteroids, ↑17-hydroxysteroids
- ↓ACTH (unless secondary to a pituitary problem)
- ↑Risk of infection, osteoporosis, psychosis

Treatment
- Adrenalectomy, removal of pituitary tumor (hypophysectomy) depending on cause
- If resulting from steroid therapy, D/C steroids slowly
- Treat complications (DM, osteoporosis)

Nursing
- Monitor for S&S
- Encourage ↓Na and altered ↑K⁺ in diet
- Protect from infection
- Teach use of medical alert band and protection from injury (fractures secondary to osteoporosis)
- Provide emotional support for altered body image and labile mood

Diabetes Mellitus (DM)

Normal glucose metabolism: Blood glucose regulated by insulin and glucagon. Insulin and glucagons are hormones. Glucose is stored as glycogen in liver and muscles or as fat in adipose tissue.
Insulin: Secreted by beta cells in islets of Langerhans in pancreas. Insulin decreases blood glucose by promoting its entry into cells.
Glucagon: Secreted by alpha cells in pancreas as blood glucose falls. Promotes release of glycogen from liver.

Etiology and Pathophysiology
■ Decreased amount of insulin or response to insulin leads to ↑blood glucose (hyperglycemia)

Type 1
■ 10% of DM; beta cell destruction ← little or no insulin for cellular metabolism of glucose; requires exogenous insulin; Type 1 DM is associated with specific human leukocyte antigens (HLA), autoantibodies, viruses. Presents at <30yr old

Type 2
■ 90% of DM; ↓sensitivity to insulin (insulin resistance) and ↓secretion of insulin; may be controlled by diet, exercise, and hypoglycemics; may need insulin when stressed; Type 2 DM is associated with obesity, genetics, inactivity, gestational diabetes. Usually presents at <45yr old

Signs and Symptoms
■ The 3 Ps: **Polyuria, Polydipsia, Polyphagia** (excessive urination, thirst, hunger)
■ Fasting blood glucose <126mg/dL, random blood glucose >200mg/dL
■ ↑Glycosylated hemoglobin (HbA1c) level indicates lack of glucose control over prior 3mo; glycosuria
■ ↓Healing
■ Type 1: ↓weight; Type 2: ↑weight

Alterations in Blood Glucose Associated with DM

Hyperglycemia	Hypoglycemia
Occurs secondary to stress, omission of medication, excess food intake; develops over days **S&S:** Polyuria; thirst; dry, hot, red skin; blurred vision; confusion; ↑P; ↓BP; S&S of dehydration	Secondary to excess insulin or oral diabetic meds, ↑exercise or ↓food while taking antidiabetic meds; develops rapidly **S&S:** Nervousness; pallor; cool, clammy skin; ↑P; tremors; slurred speech; seizure
Hyperglycemic Hyperosmolar Nonketotic Syndrome (HHNS)	**Diabetic Ketoacidosis (DKA)**
Stress (surgery, infection) and ↓insulin → severe hyperglycemia (>600mg/dL), which → polyuria and fluid shifts from cells. Results in dehydration, but not metabolic acidosis **S&S:** S&S of hyperglycemia, no ketones in urine	Stress (surgery, infection) → ↓insulin → hyperglycemia, which → glycosuria → polyuria, dehydration and breakdown of fat to meet energy needs. Excess ketones → metabolic acidosis; arterial pH <7.35 **S&S:** S&S of hyperglycemia, N&V, Kussmaul respirations, fruity breath odor, ketonuria
Somogyi Effect	**Dawn Phenomenon**
Hypoglycemia ↑release of epinephrine, corticosteroids, and GH causing rebound hyperglycemia; hyperglycemia at hs with hypoglycemia at 2:00 a.m. followed by rebound hyperglycemia in morning. Requires <insulin.	Marked increase in insulin requirements between 6:00 to 9:00 a.m. compared to midnight to 6:00 a.m. Requires >insulin.

■ **Long-term complications:**
   ■ **Microvascular changes:** Retinopathy, neuropathy, nephropathy (microalbuminuria, ↑BUN, ↑creatinine)
   ■ **Macrovascular changes:** PVD, ischemic heart disease, cerebral vascular disease

Hypothyroidism

Etiology and Pathophysiology

Primary Hypothyroidism

- Autoimmune lymphocytic destruction (**Hashimoto's thyroiditis**); secondary to toxic effect of hyperthyroidism therapy, atrophy with aging, genetics, iodides, lithium

Secondary Hypothyroidism

- Hypothalamus and/or pituitary problems ← ↑thyrotropin releasing hormone (TRH) or thyroid stimulating hormone (TSH)

Treatment

- Regular exercise to control weight and ↓insulin resistance
- ↓Calorie diet (50–60% carbohydrates, 20% protein, 20–30% fat) based on glycemic food index; ↑Soluble fiber ← slow glucose absorption
- Insulin and/or oral hypoglycemics (see Pharmacology Tab 7)
- Pancreatic or islets of Langerhans transplants
- **Treatment of DKA and HHNS:** IVF; rapid acting insulin, eventual Na and K⁺ replacement
- **Treatment of hypoglycemia:** 10–15g of simple sugar followed by complex carbohydrate and protein if conscious; glucagon injection or 50% dextrose IV if unconscious

Nursing

- Monitor S&S
- Provide foot care:
  - Inspect daily for lesions
  - Wash/dry between toes daily, wear socks and well-fitting shoes, avoid heat/cold
- Encourage weight control efforts and need for continued medical supervision (certified diabetic educator, dietician, podiatrist, ophthalmologist)
- Provide emotional support
- Teach self-monitoring of blood glucose (SMBG) and urine testing for ketones if hyperglycemic
- Teach S&S and management of hyperglycemia, hypoglycemia, and med administration
- Explain need for medical alert ID

Signs and Symptoms
- ↑Weight, lethargy, dry pale skin, brittle hair/nails
- ↓T, ↓P, ↓R, cold intolerance
- Dull expression, apathy
- Constipation, deafness, enlarged tongue, periorbital edema, anemia
- ↓T3, ↓T4, ↑TSH
- Sensitivity to CNS depressants, ↑cholesterol, ↓HDL, ↑LDL
- Severe hypothyroidism (**myxedema**) may cause coma

Treatment
- Hormone replacement with levothyroxine
- TSH levels are monitored as dose is gradually ↑ to determine optimum dose

Nursing
- Monitor S&S, ↑rest, keep warm
- Explain that symptoms will improve with hormone replacement
- Teach S&S of ↑ and ↓ thyroid function
- Teach to ↑fluids and fiber to ↓constipation
- Monitor for toxic effects of drugs (especially CNS depressants) secondary to ↓metabolism

Hyperthyroidism

Etiology and Pathophysiology
- Diffuse toxic goiter (**Graves' disease**) or autoimmune condition secondary to infection, crisis or stress. This leads to ↓thyroid-specific suppressor T-cell lymphocytes, which leads to ↑T3 (triiodothyronine) and/or ↑T4 (thyroxine). The result is an ↑metabolic rate and sensitivity to catecholamines
- Sudden severe hyperthyroidism is called **thyrotoxicosis** or **thyroid storm**
- Hyperthyroidism generally occurs between 20 and 40yr old and is more common in females

Signs and Symptoms
- ↑T, ↑P, ↑R, and ↑BP; heart failure, enlargement of gland
- Hunger, diarrhea, ↓weight
- Tremors, nervousness, bulging eyes (exophthalmos)
- Osteoporosis, amenorrhea
- ↑Sweating, flushed skin, heat intolerance
- ↑Radioactive iodine uptake, ↑T3, ↑T4, ↓TSH
- **Thyrotoxicosis**: ↑T, P >120, delirium, coma

(Continued text on following page)

Treatment
- Radioactive iodine destroys thyroid cells
- Propylthiouracil or methimazole to ↓T4
- Subtotal thyroidectomy (iodide before to ↓vascularity)

Nursing
- Monitor for S&S of thyrotoxicosis
- Provide calm, cool environment
- ↑Protein, ↑calorie diet
- Teach S&S of hypothyroidism, which may occur with treatment
- Give eye care (drops, patches) prn
- **Thyrotoxicosis:** Hypothermia blanket, oxygen, propranolol, steroids, propylthiouracil, iodide

Cardiovascular Disorders

Ischemic Heart Disease (IHD)

Etiology and Pathophysiology
- Fatty deposits in intima of coronary arteries triggers inflammatory process → plaques (atheromas) → further obstruction of blood flow → chest pain secondary to myocardial ischemia (**angina pectoris**)
- Rupture of atheroma → thrombus → severe ischemia and myocardial cell death (**myocardial infarction [MI]**)
- Other causes of MIs include ↓myocardial O_2 supply (2° vasospasm, hemorrhage) or ↑O_2 demand (2° cocaine, hyperthyroidism)

Risk Factors
- Aging, family history, race (↑African Americans), gender (males more than premenopausal females)
- HTN, diabetes mellitus, metabolic syndrome (insulin resistance, abdominal obesity, abnormal lipid profile
- Modifiable risk factors: smoking, obesity, sedentary lifestyle
- ↑Cholesterol, ↑triglycerides, ↑LDL, ↓HDL, ↑C-reactive protein (CRP)

Signs and Symptoms
Angina
- Chest pain/pressure may be substernal and/or radiate to neck, jaw, left arm
- Precipitated by exertion (↑O_2 demand), cold exposure (vasoconstriction), stress (sympathetic nervous system activity → ↑O_2 demand), heavy meal (blood diverted to GI tract → ↓blood to heart)
- Pain subsides with rest and/or nitroglycerin

Myocardial Infarction

- May have sudden chest pain (see Angina) unrelieved by rest/nitroglycerin
- SOB; restlessness; dysrhythmias
- Pulse deficit if atrial fibrillation
- Cool, pale, clammy skin; diaphoresis; N&V
- Early S&S in women: Overwhelming fatigue, dizziness, indigestion, anxiety, trouble sleeping

Diagnosis

- ECG: ↑ST segment, inverted T wave, presence of Q wave
- Echocardiogram identifies ↓ventricular wall motion and ↓ejection fraction
- ↑Myoglobin (1st to rise, but returns to normal in 12hr)
- ↑Creatine kinase (CK)
- Isoenzyme specific to heart muscle: ↑CK-MB, which ↑4-6hr after MI, ↑cardiac troponin T (cTnT) and I (cTnI), which remains ↑for 3-12hr after MI

Treatment (↓Cardiac Demands and ↑ O$_2$ to Cardiac Muscle)

Angina

- ↓Modifiable risk factors, percutaneous coronary interventional procedures (PCTA, atherectomy, stent); CABG
- Meds: nitroglycerin, beta-blockers, calcium channel blockers, antiplatelets, anticoagulants, antilipidemics
- O$_2$ prn; cardiac rehab to ↑exercise tolerance and quality of life

Myocardial Infarction

- Provide O$_2$, morphine to ↓pain, ACE inhibitors to ↓cardiac workload
- IV thrombolytic within 3hr of start of MI to dissolve clot and ↓damage
- Emergency PCI; additional care (see Angina)

Nursing

Angina

- Monitor S&S, balance activity/rest, give sublingual nitroglycerin and O$_2$ prn
- Teach about meds and to ↓modifiable risk factors

Myocardial Infarction

- Monitor S&S, ↑HOB, ↓anxiety
- Maintain IV access (avoid fluid overload)
- Identify complications (heart failure, pulmonary edema, dysrhythmias, cardiogenic shock)
- Give prescribed thrombolytic, analgesics, beta-blockers, ACE inhibitors, anticoagulants, stool softeners
- Maintain BR until stable

(Continued text on following page)

Hypertension (HTN)

Etiology and Pathophysiology
↑Systolic (SBP) and/or ↑diastolic (DBP)
Prehypertension: SBP 120-139, DBP 80-89
Stage 1: SBP 140-159, DBP 90-99
Stage 2: SBP > 160, DBP >100; ↑peripheral resistance, ↑cardiac output, and/or ↑blood volume secondary to ↑renin, ↑angiotensin, ↑aldosterone, Na retention, ↑SNS activity, pregnancy, meds, renal disease; HTN → vascular changes → ventricular hypertrophy, heart failure, MI, kidney disease, retinopathy
Preload: Stretch of cardiac muscle fibers at end of diastole
Afterload: Resistance to ejection of blood from left ventricle

Treatment
- Lifestyle modifications (see Nursing)
- Meds such as diuretics, beta-blockers, alpha-blockers, ACE inhibitors, angiotensin II receptor blockers, calcium channel blockers, vasodilators, antilipidemics

Nursing
- Monitor BP and S&S of target organ damage (SOB, angina, ↓vision, epistaxis, headache, edema)
- Teach med compliance, ↓smoking, ↓weight, ↓alcohol intake, ↑aerobic activity, ↓stress
- Teach Dietary Approaches to Stop Hypertension (**DASH**), which promotes ↓saturated fats, ↓cholesterol, ↓total fats, ↑fat dairy, and ↑in fruits, vegetables, whole grains, fish, poultry, nuts

---

- **Percutaneous transluminal coronary angioplasty (PCTA)**
- Monitor for bleeding restlessness, back pain due to retroperitoneal bleed, ↑P, ↓BP, ↑Hgb/Hct)
- Apply pressure to insertion site, keep hip extended
- Assess pulses of distal extremity
- **Postoperative coronary artery bypass graft (CABG)**
- Monitor hemodynamic status, which may be ↑ (due to heart failure or fluid overload) or ↓ (due to fluid deficit or bleeding)
- Assess pulses below vein harvest site
- Monitor ECG for dysrhythmias
- Assess urine output (if <30mL/hr, may indicate ↓renal perfusion)
- Monitor electrolytes and coagulation profile
- Maintain chest tube drainage and ventilator as needed, then encourage incentive spirometer, splinting, coughing, and deep breathing
- Provide for alternate communication while intubated
- Provide pain control
- Refer to cardiac rehab and Mended Hearts Club

Heart Failure (HF)

Etiology and Pathophysiology
- Cardiac output insufficient due to ↓ventricular filling (**diastolic HF**) or ↓ventricular contraction (**systolic HF**) → ↑SNS → ↑cardiac workload and ventricular hypertrophy → ↓renal perfusion → renin/angiotensin response → vasoconstriction and ↑aldosterone → Na and H_2O retention → ↑cardiac workload
- May → ↑pressure in pulmonary circulation (**left-sided HF**) or in the systemic circulation (**right-sided HF**)
- Severe HF may cause pulmonary edema and/or cardiogenic shock

Risk Factors
- Coronary artery disease; infection of cardiac structures
- Structural disorders of valves (mitral regurgitation, aortic stenosis)
- Dysrhythmias (rapid atrial fibrillation)
- ↑Cardiac demands related to HTN, anemia, thyrotoxicosis, fever, obesity, excessive alcohol intake

Signs and Symptoms
- ↑P, ↑R, fatigue, dyspnea, restlessness, confusion, 3rd heart sound (ventricular gallop), cardiomegaly, ↓urine
- **Signs of systemic circulation congestion:** Ankle edema, anorexia, nausea, hepatomegaly, ascites, jugular vein distention
- **Signs of pulmonic circulation congestion:** Crackles, cyanosis, frothy sputum

Diagnostic Tests
- Echocardiogram, chest x-ray (cardiomegaly), ↑brain natriuretic peptide (BNP), ↑N-terminal prohormone (NT-proBNP)

Treatment
- Treat cause (PTCA for IHD), O_2, ventricular pacing
- ACE inhibitors to ↓preload and ↓afterload
- Beta-blockers to counteract SNS overstimulation
- Diuretics to ↓fluid overload; digoxin to ↑cardiac output
- **Acute heart failure:** Intubation, mechanical ventilation, and PEEP (↓hypoxia); diuretics; morphine; dobutamine to ↑cardiac output

Nursing
- Monitor S&S; daily weight; breath sounds
- Support smoking cessation; ↓weight; gradually ↑exercise
- ↓Na diet; ↑potassium intake (dried fruit, bananas, oranges, melon)
- ↑HOB to ↓venous return; give O_2; teach about meds

Anemia

| Anemia |

Features common to all types of anemia:

Etiology and Pathophysiology
↑↓RBCs secondary to blood loss, ↓production or ↑destruction of RBCs; ↓O₂ carrying capacity of blood; ↑cardiac workload, heart failure

Signs and Symptoms
↑P, ↑R, fatigue, weakness, pallor, confusion, ↓Hgb, ↓Hct

Treatment
Correct cause, provide O₂, administer transfusions (whole blood, packed RBCs), administer meds depending on type

Nursing
Monitor S&S, balance rest/activity, ↑protein diet, teach iron supplements will cause black stools and constipation; packed red blood cells if ordered

Microcytic Anemia
■ **Etiology and pathophysiology:** ↓iron secondary to ↓dietary intake (vegetarians, teens); blood loss from GI bleeding (ulcers, cancer, inflammation) or menorrhagia; ↓iron absorption after gastric surgery
■ **Signs and symptoms:** MCV <80fl; ↓ferritin; ↑serum iron; ↑transferrin; inflammation of tongue (glossitis) and lip (cheilitis); craving for ice, clay, starch, etc. (pica)
■ **Treatment:** Oral iron best absorbed with ↓pH (give with vitamin C between meals); use straw with liquid iron (stains teeth); ↑dietary sources of iron (raisins), eggs, meat [liver], green vegetables)

Macrocytic Anemia
■ **Etiology and pathophysiology:** ↓Folate due to ↓dietary intake; alcohol; B₁₂ deficiency due to lack of intrinsic factor (pernicious anemia); ↓folate absorption after gastric surgery or Crohn's disease
■ **Signs and symptoms:** MCV >100fl; ↓folate; ↓B₁₂ (Schilling Test for pernicious anemia): sore, smooth, red, tongue; diarrhea; neuro changes due to ↓myelin (paresthesias, ataxia); screen for stomach Ca
■ **Treatment:** Oral folic acid; avoid alcohol; IM B₁₂; ↑dietary sources of folic acid (green vegetables, liver, mushrooms)

Normocytic Anemia
■ **Etiology and pathophysiology:**
■ **Hemolytic anemia (HA):** RBCs break down rapidly ← ↑release of reticulocytes; examples: sickle cell anemia, toxins, thalassemia, G-6-PD deficiency
■ **Anemia in renal disease:** ↓erythropoietin ← ↑RBC synthesis

176

- **Signs and symptoms:** MCV 80-100fl; HA → ↑reticulocytes; jaundice due to Hgb breakdown; hepatomegaly; sickle cell vaso-occlusive crisis → tissue hypoxia, necrosis, pain
  Acute hemolysis: ↑T, chills, abdominal and back pain, hemoglobinuria
  Treatment: *Sickle cell anemia:* bone marrow transplant, hydroxyurea
  Sickle cell crisis: Analgesic, hydration, O_2
  Renal disease: Iron, folate, recombinant erythropoietin

Aplastic Anemia

- **Etiology and pathophysiology:** Bone marrow stem cells destroyed → ↓RBCs, ↓WBCs (neutropenia) and ↓platelets (thrombocytopenia); idiopathic or caused by radiation, infection, or chemicals
- **Signs and symptoms:** MCV >100fl; no reticulocytes; ↓WBCs, ↓platelets; infection; bleeding (purpura, retinal hemorrhage)
- **Treatment:** Bone marrow transplant; peripheral blood stem cell transplant; immunosuppressants (cyclosporine)

Arterial Insufficiency

Etiology and Pathophysiology

- Atherosclerosis → ischemia of extremities (↑incidence in distal legs); ↓sensation → ↑risk of injury

Risk Factors

- ↑Age, males, heredity, smoking, obesity
- Inactivity, HTN, hyperlipidemia, diabetes

Signs and Symptoms

- Leg pain when walking relieved by rest (**intermittent claudication**)
- Cool, pale, shiny leg with faint/absent pulse
- ↓Hair; thick yellow toenails, toe ulcer, gangrene

Treatment

- ↓Risk factors
- Meds to ↓platelet aggregation and ↑flow
- Bypass grafts

Nursing

- Assess S&S
- Position legs ↓than heart
- Apply warmth to abdomen, local heat if ordered
- Teach to ↓ smoking, ↓ cold exposure and constrictive clothing
- **Foot care:** Inspect and protect feet, wear shoes and socks, dry feet well; dressings as ordered

Aortic Aneurysm

Etiology and Pathophysiology
- Weakness in vessel → protrusion and possible rupture

Risk Factors
- Atherosclerosis, trauma, congenital weakness, infection, inflammation
- HTN, smoking

Signs and Symptoms
- May be symptom-free; may be able to palpate a pulsating mass
- **Dissecting aneurysm:** Sudden severe chest pain extending to back, shoulder, epigastrium, abdomen; diaphoresis; ↑P

Treatment
- Confirm diagnosis with CT, MRI, sonogram
- Repair with graft
- ↑BP with antihypertensives to ↓risk of rupture or extension

Nursing
- Monitor BP, Hgb/Hct
- Assess for sudden ↑pain (may signal impending rupture)
- Teach to avoid activities that ↑intra-abdominal pressure (sneezing, coughing, vomiting, straining at stool)

Deep Vein Thrombosis

Etiology and Pathophysiology
- Virchow's triad: Venous stasis, damage to vein, ↓blood coagulation

Risk Factors
- ↑Age, obesity, immobility, oral contraceptives
- Varicose veins, popliteal pressure, fractures

Signs and Symptoms
- Edema, ache, calf pain on foot dorsiflexion (Homan's sign)
- ↑P, dyspnea, chest pain if thrombus dislodges → pulmonary embolism

Treatment
- Meds: Thrombolytic, anticoagulants
- Thrombectomy, insertion of vena cava filter to prevent PE

Nursing
- **Prevention:** Antiembolism stockings, sequential compression device, exercise, ↑fluids; prophylactic anticoagulant
- **Acute phase:** BR, ↑extremity, warm soaks if ordered

Venous Insufficiency

Etiology and Pathophysiology
- Incompetent valves and ↑venous pressure → vein dilation; ↓sensation → ↑risk of injury

Risk Factors
- Varicose veins, thrombophlebitis
- Aging, inactivity (lack of muscle contraction)

Signs and Symptoms
- Leg edema, pain, fatigue, and heaviness that ↑over day
- Brownish pigmentation of legs
- Stasis dermatitis → ankle and lower leg ulcers
- Venous ulcers more common and have more exudate than arterial ulcers

Treatment
- Positioning and supportive devices to ↓venous pressure
- Surgical and nonsurgical debridement of necrotic tissue

Nursing
- Elevate legs, apply elastic stockings before legs are dependent, avoid constrictive clothing
- Foot care: see arterial insufficiency for foot care

Respiratory Disorders

Features common to most respiratory disorders:

Etiology and Pathophysiology
- ↓Ventilation secondary to obstruction or ↓surface area for gas exchange
- Results in ↓O_2 (hypoxia) and ↑CO_2 (hypercapnia) → respiratory acidosis (↑$PaCO_2$, ↓arterial pH)

Signs and Symptoms
- ↑P, ↑ R, fatigue, weakness, restlessness, confusion
- Adventitious breath sounds, dyspnea, orthopnea, use of accessory respiratory muscles, ↓pulse oximetry

Treatment
- Based on cause, O_2, prophylactic influenza vaccine for those at ↑risk

Nursing
- Monitor S&S, ↑HOB; administer O_2, administer meds
- Teach to balance activity/rest, quit smoking

Pneumonia

Etiology and Pathophysiology
- Microorganisms from upper airway/blood, aspiration of food/gastric contents → inflammation (exudate and WBCs into alveoli) → consolidation, ↓ventilation, and ↓diffusion
- Aerosolized or droplet transmission

Risk Factors
- ↓Age, smoking, immunosuppression
- Winter (Streptococcal pneumonia), summer and fall (Legionella)

Signs and Symptoms
- ↑↑T and WBC, adventitious breath sounds, cough, sputum (character depends on organism)
- Chest x-ray indicates patchy or lobe consolidation or infiltrates

Treatment
- Antibiotic regime based on organism
- Replace fluid losses secondary to ↑T and ↑R

Nursing
- Chest PT, if ordered; ↑fluids
- Teach ↓transmission (hand washing, tissue disposal)
- Teach need to finish med regime to ↑recurrence or resistance

Tuberculosis (TB)

Etiology and Pathophysiology
- *Mycobacterium tuberculosis* → granulomas of bacilli that become fibrous tissue mass (Ghon tubercle) that can calcify or ulcerate and free bacilli
- **Miliary TB:** Bacilli may travel to bone, kidneys, or brain

Risk Factors
- ↓Immune response (HIV, steroids), crowded living conditions
- Alcoholism, malnutrition

Signs and Symptoms
- Night sweats, ↓weight, cough, hemoptysis
- +PPD/Mantoux of 10mm induration indicates immune response
- +Chest x-ray, acid fast bacteria in sputum

Treatment
- Combination of antituberculars for 6–12mo
- Prophylactic INH for exposure

Nursing
- Use airborne precautions during active disease
- Teach need for long-term compliance with meds

Emphysema

Etiology and Pathophysiology
- Alveolar wall distention → ↑surface area for gas exchange, air trapping, and ↑residual volume → ↑work to exhale, barrel chest, chronic hypercapnia; may → right-sided heart failure (**cor pulmonale**)

Risk Factors
- ↑Age, smoking, secondhand smoke, inhaled pollutants
- Alpha antitrypsin deficiency

Signs and Symptoms
- Barrel chest, clubbing of fingers
- Pursed-lip breathing, ↓forced expiratory volume
- Bronchodilators ineffective (unlike asthma)

Treatment
- Smoking cessation
- O_2; meds: steroids and bronchodilators
- Lung transplant

Nursing
- Give O_2 at ≤2L because with emphysema excessive exogenous O_2 diminishes the respiratory drive and results in ↓breathing and ↑CO_2 retention (CO_2 narcosis). Normally ↑CO_2 stimulates breathing. With emphysema there is chronic ↑CO_2 and as a result low O_2 stimulates breathing
- Teach diaphragmatic and pursed-lip breathing to extend exhalation and keep alveoli open

Lung Cancer

Etiology and Pathophysiology
- Altered DNA → alters cellular replication; may be primary or metastatic; often metastasizes to lymph nodes, bone, brain before diagnosis
- Types: Adenocarcinoma, small cell (oat cell), large cell (undifferentiated), and squamous cell carcinoma

Risk Factors
- Smoking, heredity, ↓intake of fruits and vegetables
- Exposure to asbestos or radon

(Continued text on following page)

MEDSURG

Signs and Symptoms
- Dry, chronic cough; hoarseness
- ↓Weight, lymphadenopathy
- Sputum positive for cytology
- Chest x-ray indicates lesion and possible effusion
- Biopsy indicates source (primary or secondary)

Treatment
- Lobectomy, pneumonectomy
- Chemotherapy, radiation, palliative care (↓pain)

Nursing
- Lobectomy: Manage chest tubes
- Pneumonectomy: Place on operative side
- Chemotherapy: Manage side effects; hospice prn

Acute Respiratory Distress Syndrome (ARDS)

Etiology and Pathophysiology
- Direct or indirect lung trauma → inflammation → fluid movement into alveolar spaces and ↓surfactant → atelectasis → hypoxia and ↑dead space
- Secondary to trauma, aspiration, shock, infection

Signs and Symptoms
- Early: Dyspnea, anxiety, ↓O_2 sat, ↓PaO_2
- Late: ↑CO_2, cyanosis, lung infiltrate on x-ray

Treatment
- Treat cause; mechanical ventilation and positive end expiratory pressure (PEEP—keeps alveoli open)
- Steroids, interleukin-1 receptor antagonists, surfactant therapy
- Sedatives or neuromuscular blocks to ↓"fighting" ventilator

Nursing
- Monitor S&S; suction airway
- Mechanical ventilator care:
  - Assess breath sounds for equality (PEEP → ↑risk of pneumothorax, ET tube may be in right bronchi)
  - Maintain trach or endotracheal tube cuff pressure seal to ensure full volume delivery
  - Check ventilator settings and alarms (↑pressure secondary to mucus or tubing kinks and ↓pressure secondary to ↓cuff pressure or separation of tubing)
  - Provide alternate mode of communication

Pneumothorax

- Disruption of lining of lung (visceral pleura) or lining of thoracic cavity (parietal pleura) permitting air (pneumothorax) and/or blood (hemothorax) into pleural space → lung collapse
- 2° rib fx, stab or gunshot wound, thoracentesis, emphysema

Signs and Symptoms
- Sudden unilateral chest pain
- ↑P, ↑R, dyspnea, ↓breath sounds on affected side, ↓PaO$_2$
- Air/blood in pleural space on x-ray

Treatment
- O$_2$, assist with insertion of chest tube/water seal drainage to reestablish negative pressure (pneumothorax—2nd anterior intercostal space, hemothorax—lower and more posterior space)

Nursing
- Monitor S&S; relieve pain
- Assess water seal chamber fluid level (↑ on inspiration and ↓ with exhalation) and for bubbling in water seal chamber (continuous bubbling suggests air leak and absence suggests full lung expansion or blocked tube)
- Instruct patient to exhale and bear down when removing chest tube, then apply occlusive dressing
- **Subcutaneous emphysema**: Palpate around insertion site for crackles, which indicates air in subcutaneous tissue (crepitus)

Musculoskeletal Disorders

Fractures

Break in bone continuity from excessive force. Traumatizes muscles, blood vessels, and nerves leading to inflammation and possible hemorrhage

Types of Fractures
Simple (closed): Skin remains intact
Compound (open): Fragments penetrate skin
Transverse: Straight across
Oblique: Angled across
Spiral: Twists around shaft
Comminuted: Multiple fragments
Compression: Compressed bone mass
Depressed: Fragments forced inward

(Continued text on following page)

Green stick: Break partially extends across and then along length; more common in children

Pathological: <Force than normal needed to break bone due to ↑age, porous, brittle bones (osteoporosis), metastatic or primary tumors, Paget's disease

Signs and Symptoms

- Pain, spasms, shortening of extremity, ecchymosis
- Grating sound when moved (crepitus)
- ↓Mobility, deformity, paresthesia 2° nerve damage
- Shock 2° hemorrhage
- **Fat emboli:** Dyspnea; ↑R; ↑P; ↑T; copious white sputum; crackles; ↑mentation; buccal, conjunctival and chest petechiae
- **Compartment syndrome:** ↑Muscle compartment pressure 2° edema/bleeding → ↓circulation → tissue hypoxia → ↑pain and damage

Treatment

- Closed reduction: Fragments aligned and stabilized with cast, splint, or traction
- Open reduction and internal fixation (ORIF) with wires, pins, nails, rods, or plates
- Hemiarthroplasty (surgery for femur head prosthesis)

Nursing

- Immobilize (↓trauma and pain); pain management
- **Peripheral neurovascular assessment:** Peripheral pulses, color, T, capillary refill, motor/sensory function
- Monitor for compartment syndrome (elevate limb and notify MD)
- **Patient with a cast:** ↑On pillow, uncover to ↑drying, handle with palms not fingertips until dry, isometric exercise to ↓atrophy; odor may indicate infection
- **Patient with traction:** Hang weights freely, functional alignment, pin care as ordered for skeletal traction
- **Postoperative care for patient with hemiarthroplasty:**
  - ↓Pain (patient controlled analgesia)
  - ↓Displacement of prosthesis (abduction pillow, avoid internal rotation or flexing >90°, ↑toilet seat/chair)
  - Prevent DVT (anticoagulants and compression devices as ordered, dorsiflexion, avoid popliteal pressure)
  - ↓Atelectasis/pneumonia (incentive spirometry, coughing, deep breathing)

Arthritis

Rheumatoid Arthritis (RA)	Osteoarthritis (OA)	Gouty Arthritis
Immune response → inflammation, breakdown of collagen, synovial edema, pannus formation, narrowed joint space, bone spurs **Risk factors:** ↑in female	Involves chondrocyte response → cartilage breakdown **Risk factors:** ↑Age, obesity, joint injury, repetitive use, congenital hip subluxation	Purine metabolism defect → ↑serum uric acid → urate deposits that become porous stone (**tophi**) **Risk factors:** Starvation, organ meat and shellfish intake, ↑cell proliferation (leukemia, psoriasis), ↑ in males
S&S: Acute bilateral inflammation of joints (hands, wrists, feet, and later other joints). Pain unrelieved by rest. AM stiffness >1hr. Deformities (ulnar drift, swan neck). ↑ESR ↑C-reactive protein, ↑rheuma-toid factor, ↑ANA. Synovial fluid has narrowed joint spaces, enlarged joints, tender complements and ↑WBCs. Fatigue, anemia, ↑T, ↑node size	**S&S:** Morning stiffness of hips, knees, cervical/lumbar spine, small joints of hands and feet for <1 hr; improves with activity. Enlargement of distal interphalangeal finger joints (**Heberden nodes**). If inflamed, narrowed joint spaces, tender joint movement	**S&S:** Acute asymmetric joint pain and inflammation. Located most often in big toe but may affect ankle, knee, elbow, wrist or fingers. Tophi in periphery (outer ear, feet, hands, elbows, knees). ↑Serum uric acid, uric acid crystals in synovial fluid, urate renal calculi and nephropathy
Treatment: Meds, including steroids, NSAIDs, COX-2 inhibitors, antirheumatic drugs (DMARDs). Surgery: joint fusion, joint replacement, or synovectomy	**Treatment:** Meds, including acetaminophen, COX-2 inhibitors, glucosamine and chondroitin, topical capsaicin; knee-joint injections of hyaluronic acid; arthroplasty	**Treatment:** Meds, including colchicine, probenecid, allopurinol. ↓Intake of purines (organ meats) and alcohol. ↑Fluid intake to ↓renal calculi

Nursing: Balance rest/activity, provide or teach ROM. Joints in functional alignment, heat or cold as ordered. Administer meds and provide non-drug pain relief measures. ↓Weight prn. Adaptive devices to ↑independence. Refer to Arthritis Foundation.

Chronic Neurological Disorders

Multiple Sclerosis

Etiology and Pathophysiology
- Autoimmune response → demyelination of CNS neurons and formation of sclerotic plaques → ↓impulse conduction
- Remissions and exacerbations with downward plateaus
- S&S vary depending on nerves involved

Risk Factors
- Caucasian race 20-40yr old
- Female gender

Signs and Symptoms
- Charcot's triad (intention tremor, nystagmus, scanning speech)
- Visual disturbances (diplopia, visual field deficits)
- Fatigue, paresthesias of face and/or extremities, incoordination, slurred speech, spasticity
- Bladder dysfunction

Treatment
- Disease modifying therapy (interferon beta-1a and -1b, glatiramer acetate)
- Meds: Corticosteroids, antispasmodics (baclofen)
- Palliative care

Nursing
- Monitor S&S, balance activity/rest, provide cool environment, ↓fat diet
- Safe mobility: Wide base of support, assistive devices
- ↓Pressure ulcers: Change position q1-2hr, skin care, pull sheet to ↓shearing, pressure relieving devices
- Improve elimination pattern: Respond to urge, follow bowel and bladder toileting schedule, ↑fiber and fluids, ascorbic acid to acidify urine if ordered
- Emotional support: ↑Ventilation of feelings, refer to National Multiple Sclerosis Society

Seizures

Etiology and Pathophysiology
■ Sudden, abnormal electrical discharge from cerebral neurons → generalized seizures (affect both hemispheres) or partial seizure (start in one area of the brain)
■ Secondary to cerebral vascular disease, head trauma, brain tumor, drug or alcohol withdrawal, hypoglycemia, ↑T in children

Signs and Symptoms of Generalized Seizures
■ **Tonic-clonic seizures** (formerly grand mal seizure):
  ■ Intense muscle contractions (tonic phase), alternating with muscle relaxation (clonic phase)
  ■ Often preceded by aura (flash of light, special noise)
  ■ Unconsciousness, shallow/absent breathing, bladder/bowel incontinence
  ■ Confusion, drowsiness, and/or sleep following seizure
■ **Absence seizure** (formerly petit mal seizure):
  ■ Abrupt, brief (3-5sec) loss of consciousness
  ■ More common in children; may disappear at puberty
■ **Myoclonic seizure:**
  ■ Short (few min), sporadic periods of muscle contractions; rare
  ■ Often secondary seizures
■ **Febrile seizure:**
  ■ Tonic-clonic seizure with T>101.8°F; most common in children
  ■ Self-limiting
■ **Status epilepticus:**
  ■ Continuous tonic-clonic seizure activity for >30min
  ■ Medical emergency; IV benzodiazepines

Signs and Symptoms of Partial (Focal) Seizure
■ **Simple:**
  ■ Single muscle movement (twitch) or sensory alteration
  ■ ↑Alkaline phosphatase
■ **Complex** (formerly psychomotor or temporal lobe seizure):
  ■ Complex sensory, motor, or autonomic response with altered LOC
  ■ May be preceded by aura
  ■ Associated with blank stare, lack of attention to verbal stimuli, and chewing, swallowing, fumbling movements
  ■ Usually onset occurs in late adolescence
  ■ No memory of event following seizure

(Continued text on following page)

Parkinson's Disease

Etiology and Pathophysiology
- Neuronal destruction of substantia nigra in basal ganglia → ↑dopamine → neurotransmitter imbalance; progressive degeneration

Risk Factors
- Genetics, male gender, 50–60yr old, atherosclerosis

Signs and Symptoms
- Resting tremor (pill-rolling motion of thumb against fingers)
- Shuffling gait, no arm swing; slow voluntary movement (bradykinesia)
- Stooped posture, masklike facies, rigidity, monotone voice, dysphagia, constipation, incontinence

Treatment
- Anti-Parkinson agents, anticholinergics, antivirals, dopamine agonist, MAO inhibitors
- Deep brain stimulation
- Destruction of thalamus for tremor and globus pallidus for bradykinesia

Nursing
- Maintain airway, balance activity and rest
- Safe mobility: Wide base of support, assistive devices, concentration to walk erect
- Body movement: Warm baths and active ROM to ↑rigidity; splints to ↑contractures
- Bowel elimination: ↑Fluids, ↑roughage, use raised toilet seat
- Nutrition: Assistive devices, bite-size pieces, thickened liquids
- Emotional support: ↑Ventilation of feelings, refer to National Parkinson's Foundation

Treatment
- Antiseizure agents
- Treat underlying cause (e.g., antipyretic)

Nursing
- Identify presence of status epilepticus
- Monitor S&S before, during, and after seizure
- Protect patient (ease to floor if out of bed, protect head, loosen clothes, avoid insertion of airway when jaw is clenched, avoid restraining, lateral position if possible)
- Teach need to adhere to antiseizure therapy to maintain therapeutic levels, continue follow-up, wear medical alert band
- Emotional support, refer to Epilepsy Foundation of America

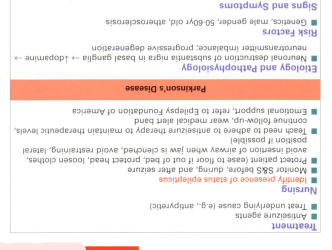

Neurological Disorders With Respiratory Insufficiency

Myasthenia Gravis	Guillain-Barré Syndrome	Amyotrophic Lateral Sclerosis (ALS; Lou Gehrig's Disease)
Autoimmune response → antibody attachment to acetylcholine receptor sites causing destruction of acetylcholine → ↓impulse transmission → ↓ muscle weakness that worsens with activity and improves with rest **Risk factors:** Females, 20–40yr old; males, 60–70yr old **S&S:** Double vision (**diplopia**), eyelid droop (**ptosis**), snarl (**myasthenic smile**), voice change (**dysphonia**) **Myasthenic crisis:** General weakness, aphagia, respiratory failure **Treatment:** Anticholinesterase agents (neostigmine, pyridostigmine); plasmapheresis; steroids; thymectomy to ↓antibodies	Autoimmune response → ascending destruction → ↓ability to transmit impulses; often occurs a few wk after infection; Schwann cells eventually produce myelin → recovery, but may take 2yr and leave residual deficits **Risk factors:** Vaccination, infection, pregnancy **S&S:** Ascending symmetrical weakness/paralysis, areflexia and paresthesia; respiratory paralysis; aphagia; autonomic nerve dysfunction → labile P and BP rates **Treatment:** IgG IV, O₂, plasmapheresis, tracheostomy and mechanical ventilation, prevent complications of immobility (anticoagulants)	Cause unknown; possible autoimmune response or excess nerve stimulation by glutamate → progressive loss of upper and lower motor neurons → lack of muscle stimulation → progressive atrophy; life expectancy about 3–5yr **Risk factors:** Males, 50–60yr old **S&S:** Fatigue, weakness, impaired coordination, muscle twitching (**fasciculations**), nasal-sounding voice, ↑deep tendon reflexes, dysarthria, dysphagia, dyspnea **Treatment:** Riluzole (a glutamate antagonist) may prolong life, antispasmodics (baclofen), enteral feedings, ventilation

Nursing: Myasthenia Gravis, Guillain-Barré, Amyotrophic Lateral Sclerosis

- Monitor S&S, particularly respiratory status
- Support respirations: O₂; Fowler's position, suctioning, chest PT; incentive spirometer; maintain ET tube, tracheostomy, mechanical ventilator if present
- Prevent pulmonary embolus: ROM, prevent popliteal pressure, use sequential compression devices on legs as ordered
- Prevent pressure ulcers: Reposition q1–2hr, skin care, pull sheet to ↓shearing, use pressure relieving devices
- Support nutrition: Assess weight, assist with oral intake and prevent aspiration (↑HOB, feed slowly, use thickening product), provide parenteral or enteral feedings if ordered
- Provide emotional support: Recognize LOC and mental status are not affected but may be unable to speak
- Devise alternate means of communication
- Refer to MG Foundation, GB Foundation, or ALS Association
- Myasthenia Gravis:
- Distinguish between myasthenic and cholinergic crises: both cause respiratory muscle weakness, inability to swallow (aphagia), and difficulty speaking (dysarthria)
- Giving ordered edrophonium (rapid-acting anticholinesterase) improves symptoms of myasthenic crisis and intensifies symptoms of cholinergic crisis
- Administer meds at precise times and schedule meals at peak action; provide rest periods

Brain Attack (BA)/Cerebrovascular Accident (CVA)

Etiology and Pathophysiology
- Irreversible neurological deficit caused by cerebral ischemia 2° embolus, thrombus, hemorrhage (subarachnoid or intracerebral bleeding)

Risk Factors
- Transient ischemic attack (TIA) in which deficits last <24hr may precede BA
- ↑Age, male gender, ↑BP, DM, cardiac disease, hyperlipidemia
- ↑African American heritage, obesity, smoking, oral contraceptives

Signs and Symptoms
- Based on location/extent of damage
- ↑Intracranial pressure (ICP): Headache, restlessness, ↓LOC, ↑systolic BP and widening pulse pressure, ↑T, ↓P, ↑R, vomiting, vision problems, unilateral pupil changes, seizures, posturing—arms extended and turned in (decerebrate) or arms flexed, legs internally rotated (decorticate)

- **Motor:** Weakness (**hemiparesis**) or paralysis (**hemiplegia**) on side of body opposite to affected side of brain; difficulty swallowing (**dysphagia**)
- **Bowel/bladder:** Constipation; frequency, urgency; incontinence
- **Sensory:** Unilateral paresthesia, loss of $1/2$ visual field (**hemianopsia**), ↓proprioception
- **Communication:** ↓Articulation (**dysarthria**), difficulty communicating thoughts in words (**expressive, Broca's aphasia**), difficulty understanding communication (**receptive, Wernicke's aphasia**)
- **Cognitive/emotional:** Lability of mood, ↓memory, ↓attention span, ↓judgment

Treatment

- **Acute phase:**
    - Thrombolytic therapy with tissue plasminogen activator (t-PA) within 3hr and anticoagulants for ischemic BA
    - Steroids to ↓ICP secondary to cerebral edema
    - PT, OT, speech therapy
    - NGT feedings
- **Rehabilitation phase:** Multidisciplinary depending on needs
- **Prevention:**
    - ↓Weight, ↓fat diet, smoking cessation
    - Antihypertensives for HTN, anticoagulant for AF, glucose control for DM
    - Carotid endarterectomy

Nursing

- Monitor S&S, balance activity/rest, semi-Fowler's to ↓ICP
- Seizure precautions
- Prevent aspiration: Suction, positioning, thicken liquids or enteral tube feedings
- Maintain mobility/prevent contractures: ROM, position changes, splints
- Prevent thrombophlebitis: Anticoagulants, ↓popliteal pressure, ROM, sequential compression devices on legs
- Prevent pressure ulcers: Position change q1-2hr, skin care, pull sheet to ↓shearing, pressure relieving devices
- Promote communication: Use picture board; simple sentences with visual clues for receptive aphasia; have patience and avoid completing patient's message for expressive aphasia
- Support elimination: Respond immediately to urge; bowel and bladder training
- Provide emotional support: Involve with planning, accept emotional lability and expressions of grieving for losses

Spinal Cord Injury

Etiology and Pathophysiology
- Injury secondary to contusion, compression, laceration, transection
- Edema and bleeding → ischemia → ↑injury
- Frequently affects C5-7, T12-L1

Risk Factors
- <30yr old, male gender
- MVAs, violence, falls, diving, contact sports, tumors

Signs and Symptoms
- Level of injury determines S&S
- **Spinal shock:** Flaccid paralysis, loss of sensation and reflexes below injury, loss of bowel and bladder function
- **Neurogenic shock:** ↓BP, ↓P, inability to sweat; secondary to ↓autonomic nerve activity
- **Paralysis:** Depends on level of injury—all 4 extremities is called *quadriplegia*, paralysis of legs only is called *paraplegia*
- **Bladder dysfunction:**
  - **Spastic bladder:** Empties automatically when detrusor muscle is stretched; occurs with injury above conus medullaris
  - **Flaccid bladder:** Atonic bladder distends and periodically overflows but does not empty; occurs with injury at or below conus medullaris
- **Autonomic hyperreflexia:**
  - Exaggerated SNS response with cord injury ≥T6
  - Mainly secondary to bladder or bowel distention
  - Headache, ↑BP, ↓P, "goose bumps" (**piloerection**), nasal congestion, diaphoresis, nausea
- **Respiratory paralysis:** Lack of voluntary breathing with injury above C3-4

Treatment
- Stabilize head, neck, and spine on backboard for transport
- MRI to assess injury
- IV corticosteroids to ↓cerebral edema
- Respiratory support secondary to paralyzed or weak intercostals
- Surgery: ↓Compression, correct alignment and ↑spine stability
- Traction with skeletal tongs or halo device
- NGT for gastric decompression secondary to paralytic ileus
- Urinary retention catheter to ↓bladder distention
- Multidisciplinary rehabilitation (RT, PT, OT, vocational education)

Nursing

- Identify and treat autonomic hyperreflexia: ↑HOB, loosen clothing, avoid cutaneous stimulation, ensure empty bladder, catheterize to ↓urinary distention prn, remove fecal mass after application of anesthetic ointment prn
- Use American Spinal Injury Association (ASIA) scale to determine extent of motor and sensory dysfunction
- Assess R, pulse oximetry, ABGs; encourage coughing, deep breathing, hydration; chest PT
- Prevent DVT and PE: monitor calf and thigh circumference, give ordered anticoagulants, use sequential compression devices, avoid popliteal pressure or calf massage
- ↓Spasticity and prevent contractures: ROM, splints to ↓footdrop, trochanter rolls to ↓external hip rotation, give ordered antispasmodics
- Maintain skin integrity: position changes (teach patient to shift weight if possible); hygiene; massage; special bed, mattress, chair cushion; ↑protein and vitamin C in diet
- Provide pin site care—cleanse with ordered solution, apply topical antibiotic
- Digital stimulation of rectum after meal can promote defecation, ↑fluids, ↑fiber, assist with bowel training
- Support urinary elimination: intermittent catheterization
- Provide emotional support: involve with planning, assist with coping with losses, discuss sexual concerns (may have reflex erection and ejaculation)

Obesity

Morbid Obesity

- 100lb >ideal body wt; ↑risk for cardiovascular disease, arthritis, asthma, bronchitis, DM, impaired body image, ↓self-esteem, depression

Treatment

- Diet, behavior modification, exercise
- Bariatric surgery if conservative treatment is unsuccessful (**gastric bypass, vertical banded gastroplasty**)
  - After surgery ↑risk for peritonitis, obstruction, atelectasis, pneumonia, thromboembolism, nutritional deficiencies, metabolic disturbances due to N&V
  - Weight gain if diet is not followed

Nursing

- Support weight loss diet modification and exercise regimen
- **Postoperative:** NPO; 6 small feedings daily as ordered (600-800 calories total) when bowel sounds return; ↑po fluids (↓dehydration); assess for bleeding, peritonitis, thromboembolism, electrolyte imbalances; teach to eat small amounts slowly or vomiting and painful esophageal distention will occur; provide emotional support (body image, dietary restrictions needs for body contouring surgery prn)

Gastrointestinal Disorders

GERD and Hiatal Hernia

Gastroesophageal Reflux Disease (GERD)
Etiology and Pathophysiology
- Gastric contents enter esophagus causing inflammation; may cause a precancerous condition **(Barrett's esophagus)**
- Secondary to ↓lower esophageal sphincter (LES) tone, obesity, hiatal hernia, pregnancy

Signs and Symptoms
- Heartburn **(pyrosis)**, hoarseness, wheezing, dysphagia
- Esophageal pH shows acidity, endoscopy or barium swallow reveal tissue damage

Treatment
- Proton pump inhibitors, H_2 receptor blockers, antacids, cholinergics
- Surgery to tighten esophageal fundus

Hiatal Hernia

Etiology and Pathophysiology
- Part of stomach slides upward into thoracic cavity; may cause reflux, obstruction, hemorrhage
- Secondary to obesity, congenital weakness, pregnancy, female gender

Signs and Symptoms
- May be asymptomatic, evident in barium swallow
- Sense of fullness, regurgitation, pyrosis, dysphagia, nocturnal dyspnea

Treatment
- Paraesophageal hernias may require emergency surgery to ↓restricted blood flow
- See GERD

Nursing Care for Hiatal Hernia and GERD
- Monitor S&S; support weight control
- Teach patient to have small, frequent, low-fat meals; drink fluids between meals; and remain upright 1hr after meals
- Teach patient to ↑HOB to prevent nighttime distress
- Advise patient to avoid tight belts and waistlines and to avoid chocolate, caffeine, alcohol, and peppermint, which ↓LES tone

	Peptic Ulcer and Gastric Carcinoma			
	Etiology and Pathophysiology	Risk Factors	Signs and Symptoms	Treatment
Peptic ulcer disease	↑Pepsin, ↑HCl acid or ↓tissue resistance to acid → gastric or duodenal ulcers May → hemorrhage, perforation, or peritonitis	*Helicobacter pylori*, NSAIDs, alcohol, stress, smoking Zollinger-Ellison syndrome (↑HCl)	Gnawing epigastric pain Duodenal ulcer pain occurs 2-3hr pc and is relieved by food Gastric ulcer pain occurs <1hr pc and is relieved by vomiting	Antibiotics (*H. pylori*), proton pump inhibitors, H₂ receptor blockers Surgery: Vagotomy to ↓HCl, antrectomy, and reattachment to duodenum (Billroth I) or jejunum (Billroth II)
Gastric Carcinoma	Generally caused by adenocarcinoma which can metastasize to liver, bone, pancreas, or esophagus before diagnosis	Smoked food, pernicious anemia, gastric ulcers, *H. pylori*, Japanese descent, male gender	May be asymptomatic Anorexia, ↓weight, anemia, lack of HCl (achlorhydria), heartburn Biopsy identifies cancer cells; bone and liver scans identify metastasis	Gastrectomy Radiation, chemotherapy Tumor markers used to check progress (carcinoembryonic antigen, CA19-9, CA50)

Nursing Care for PUD and Gastric Carcinoma

- Assess VS; note amount of coffee ground or frankly bloody emesis or melena. Assess for S&S of shock
- Manage NG tube and NS lavage for bleeding
- Assess for life-threatening perforation: Life-threatening; S&S: ↑P, abdominal pain, rigid boardlike abdomen, and diaphoresis
- **Dumping syndrome:** Hypertonic gastric contents move rapidly into intestine → shift of intravascular fluid into intestine. Results in ↑P, ↓BP, diaphoresis, and fainting. Limit by teaching no fluid with meals, small frequent meals, avoiding simple carbohydrates, remaining upright 1hr after meals

Lower GI Disorders

Inflammatory Bowel Disease (IBD)		Diverticulosis and Diverticulitis	Colorectal Cancer
Regional Enteritis	**Ulcerative Colitis**		
Crohn's disease. Affects distal ileum and colon. Mucosal thickening with discrete ulcers. May → fissures, abscesses that → thick walls and narrow lumen	Affects colon and rectum. Superficial ulcerations cause edema, bleeding. Abscesses → thick walls and narrow lumen. ↑Risk of colon cancer	Pouchlike herniations through muscle layer of colon (**diverticulosis**). Trapped food or feces cause inflammation (**diverticulitis**) that may lead to bleeding, obstruction, perforation, and/or peritonitis	Adenocarcinoma of epithelial lining invades surrounding tissue by direct extension into lumen. Results in colon narrowing and ulcerations, or metastasis via blood or lymph to other sites (liver)
Risk factors: Genetics, young adults, smoking	**Risk factors:** Jewish, 30-50yr old, Caucasians	**Risk factors:** ↑Age, genetics, lack of fiber, constipation	**Risk factors:** Polyps; IBD; ↑age; genetics; ↑fat, ↓fiber, ↑protein, diet
S&S: RLQ cramping pain pc, ↑T, ↓weight, diarrhea, rectal bleeding	**S&S:** LLQ abdominal cramps, ↓weight, rectal bleeding, diarrhea	**S&S:** LLQ abdominal pain, ↑T, ↑WBC, fatigue, diarrhea or constipation	**S&S:** Diarrhea/constipation, ribbon/pencil-shaped stool, ↓weight, anemia, abdominal distention
Treatment for IBD: Antidiarrheals, antispasmodics, steroids, sulfasalazine, metronidazole. Surgery if needed: colectomy with ileoanal anastomosis, ileostomy, continent ileostomy (Kock pouch *Exacerbation:* NPO, TPN, IVF. Then rest bowel with ↓residue, ↑protein, ↑calorie diet. *Remission:* Fiber, bulk laxatives to ↓diarrhea		**Treatment:** Antispasmodics, IVF, antibiotics, and NPO for acute phase. Then ↓ residue until inflammation subsides. Dietary fiber and bulk laxative to ↓recurrence. Temporary colostomy; colon resection	**Treatment:** Surgery: may be colon resection, hemicolectomy, or abdominal/perineal resection with colostomy. Radiation. Chemotherapy and carcinoembryonic antigen to mark tumor and response to treatment.

Nursing Care for Disorders of the Lower GI Tract

- Monitor S&S and bowel sounds
  - Shape and consistency of stool
  - Presence of blood in stool (frank blood, melena)
- Support coping with disease chronicity; teach diet
- Assess for S&S of perforation/peritonitis: rigid boardlike abdomen, diaphoresis, ↑T, ↑P, ↓BP
- Surgery:
  - *Preoperative:* Provide liquid diet x 48hr, antibiotics to ↓intestinal flora, laxatives, enemas PM before surgery
  - *Postoperative:* Monitor VS, breath sounds, bowel sounds; provide pain control; nasogastric decompression until peristalsis resumes, then advance diet as tolerated; avoid gas-forming foods; IVs to maintain F&E balance; wound care (irrigations or sitz baths for hygiene, comfort, and packing removal)
  - Prevent pneumonia by teaching patient about coughing, deep breathing, incentive spirometry
  - Prevent DVT by teaching patient about ankle pumping, early ambulation. Apply sequential compression devices and avoid pressure behind the popliteal space
- For the patient with a colostomy:
  - Assess stoma: pink/brick red is normal; pale, purple, or black indicates ischemia
  - Assess bowel sounds, distention, character/amt of stool that usually begins in 3-6 days
  - Determine consistency of stool; ostomy site determines nature of stool (ileostomy constantly drains liquid stool; sigmoid colostomy stool usually is solid)
  - Apply appliance with 1/8in clearance around stoma to avoid stoma constriction or excess skin exposure to stool
  - Clean area with soap and water; use protective barrier and antifungal agent (nystatin) if ordered on skin under appliance
  - Empty appliance when $^1/_2$ full to ↓leakage
  - Irrigate distal colostomy with 105°F water at same time daily to regulate elimination
  - Refer to United Ostomy Association or enterostomal therapist

Disorders of Accessory Organs of Digestion

Cholecystitis

Etiology and Pathophysiology
- Impaired bile flow → gallbladder inflammation (**cholelithiasis**), distention, and autolysis. This leads to gangrene or perforation; blocked bile flow may → obstructive jaundice
- Usually secondary to gallstones or other precipitates

Risk Factors
- 4 Fs: fair, fat, ≥ forty, female
- Rapid ↓weight, cirrhosis
- Estrogen therapy
- Multiple pregnancies
- DM

Signs and Symptoms
- RUQ abdominal pain usually radiating to back subscapular area especially after ↑fat meal
- N&V, ↑T, rebound tenderness, obstructive jaundice evidenced by yellow skin and sclera, dark urine, and clay-colored stools
- Signs of bleeding 2° ↓fat digestion causing ↓absorption of the fat soluble vitamin K
- ↑WBC, ↑serum bilirubin, ↑alkaline phosphatase

Treatment
- Laparoscopic or abdominal removal of gallbladder (**cholecystectomy**)
- Incision into common bile duct (**choledochostomy**)
- Dissolution of stones by oral chenodiol or infusion of solvent into gallbladder

Nursing
- Monitor S&S
- Teach ↓fat diet; teach use of incentive spirometer and coughing (incision near diaphragm)
- Preoperative vitamin K, analgesics
- Maintain T-tube drainage if bile duct explored. Tube will be removed when stool regains brown color, which indicates bile flow

Hepatitis

Etiology and Pathophysiology
- Inflammation of liver secondary to infection, parasitic infestation, alcohol, toxins, drugs (INH, acetaminophen)
- **Hepatitis A (HAV)** and **E (HEV):** Spread via fecal-oral route; secondary to ↓sanitation and eating shellfish from contaminated water
- **Hepatitis B (HBV), C (HCV),** and **D (HDV):** Spread by contact with contaminated blood; secondary to sexual contact, shared sharps (needles, razors)

Risk Factors
- Health care professionals
- Multiple sexual partners
- Intravenous drug users
- Hemophiliacs due to frequent transfusions of clotting factors
- 30% have unidentifiable sources

Signs and Symptoms
- May be asymptomatic
- *Preicteric stage:* Flulike symptoms
- *Icteric stage:* N&V, anorexia, malaise, jaundice, presence of specific hepatitis antigens and antibodies; ↑aspartate aminotransferase AST, ↑alanine aminotransferase (ALT)

Treatment
- Antivirals (interferon)
- Vaccines against HAV and HBV before exposure provide active immunity
- Immune globulins provide passive immunity post exposure

Nursing
- Monitor S&S
- ↑Calories, ↑protein, ↓fat diet as ordered
- Contact precautions for HAV and HEV
- Teach to avoid toxins (acetaminophen, alcohol, carbon tetrachloride, INH)

Cirrhosis

Etiology and Pathophysiology
- Fibrous scar tissue and fat accumulate in liver →hepatomegaly and portal hypertension. Results in esophageal varices, hemorrhoids, obstructive jaundice and ascites
- ↓Liver function → ↓metabolism → ↑ammonia (a metabolized protein by-product) → encephalopathy

(Continued text on following page)

Pancreatitis

Etiology and Pathophysiology
- Obstruction of pancreatic duct causes reflux of trypsin resulting in autodigestion that leads to inflammation
- Possible necrosis with calcification, perforation, or hemorrhage
- Pancreatic pseudocysts or abscesses may develop
- May be idiopathic, acute or chronic and result in DM

Risk Factors
- Alcoholism in middle-age men, biliary disease in older females
- Extremely high triglycerides (>1000mg/dL)

Signs and Symptoms
- Epigastric pain that ↑ with eating and may radiate to thorax/back
- N&V, ↑T, ↑weight

Risk Factors
- Alcoholism (most common), hepatitis or biliary disease
- Industrial chemicals, male gender, 40-60yr old

Signs and Symptoms
- ↑Liver enzymes (AST, ALT, LDH, GGT), jaundice, hepatomegaly
- ↓Albumin, ↑bilirubin, ↓globulins, ↑ammonia, ↑PT
- Ascites, GI varices, edema secondary to ↓albumin and ↑aldosterone, which causes retention of Na and H_2O
- Confusion, agitation, flapping hand tremors (**asterixis**)
- Liver biopsy to confirm diagnosis

Treatment
- Vitamins (A, D, E, K, B), zinc, colchicine, K⁺ sparing diuretics
- Lactulose to ↓ammonia; albumin
- Portal caval shunt, sclerotherapy or balloon tamponade for varices
- Paracentesis for ascites with dyspnea

Nursing
- Monitor S&S, I&O, abdominal girth
- Teach to avoid alcohol
- **Liver biopsy:** Have patient hold breath during needle insertion; keep on right side with pillow against insertion site. Assess for bleeding
- **Paracentesis:** Have patient void before and maintain an upright position during procedure; after assess respiratory status, S&S of shock, persistent leakage
- **Balloon tamponade:** Provide oral suction, maintain traction on gastric balloon, monitor pressure of esophageal balloon

- Abdominal distention, jaundice
- Steatorrhea and glucose intolerance with chronic pancreatitis
- ↑Amylase, ↑lipase, ↓serum calcium
- S&S of perforation: Rebound tenderness, rigid abdomen, shock

Treatment
- NPO, IVF and electrolyte replacement
- NGT to ↓GI motility and ↓secretions
- Antibiotics, anticholinergics, pancreatic enzymes (lipase, trypsin, amylase) with meals for chronic pancreatitis
- Surgery if secondary to biliary disease

Nursing
- Give analgesics but avoid morphine; may ↑spasm of sphincter of Oddi
- Vitamins A and E, and ↓fat diet as ordered
- Monitor I&O, S&S of tetany and hyperglycemia
- Provide small frequent meals
- Support abstinence from alcohol; refer to Alcoholics Anonymous

Female Reproductive Cancers

Overview of Cancer

Cancer is the mutation of cellular DNA resulting in abnormal cells that invade other tissue by extension or metastasis via lymph or blood.

Types
Adenocarcinoma (glandular), carcinoma (epithelial), glioma (CNS), leukemia (blood forming), lymphoma (lymphatic), melanoma (pigmented), myeloma (plasma of bone marrow), sarcoma (soft tissue, muscle, vascular, synovial)

Risk Factors
Genetics, microbiological agents (herpes simplex virus/cervical Ca), physical agents (sun exposure/skin Ca), hormones (estrogen/breast Ca), chemical agents (smoking/lung Ca), diet (↑fat/colon Ca), ↓immune response (AIDS/Kaposi's sarcoma)

Early Detection
See CAUTION in Basic Information Tab 2. Screening: Yearly cervical pap tests at 18yr, yearly clinical breast exam and monthly SBE at 20yr, yearly mammogram at 40yr, yearly fecal occult blood test at 50yr, colonoscopy every 5-10yr at 50yr, yearly PSA and digital rectal exam at 50yr

Staging
Staging helps determine treatment and prognosis; see p. 202

TNM Staging		
Size of Tumor (T)	**Nodal Involvement (N)**	**Metastasis (M)**

TX: Not assessable
TO: No evidence of tumor
Tis: In situ
T1-4: Increasing
  tumor size
	NX: Not assessable
	NO: No metastasis to
	  regional nodes
	N1-3: Increasing regional
	  node involvement
		MX: Not assessable
		MO: No metastasis
		M1: Metastasis

General Nursing Care for Patients With Cancer

- Teach healthy lifestyle (no smoking, weight control, ↓fat diet with ↑intake of cruciferous vegetables and carotenoids, ↓sun exposure)
- Encourage routine screening; refer to American Cancer Society
- Support pain management
- Support advanced directives (living will, health care proxy)
- **Manage side effects of treatment:**
  - **Stomatitis:** Oral care (soft toothbrush/sponge toothette), avoid mouthwash with alcohol, rinse with viscous lidocaine ac as prescribed, ↓spicy or extreme temperatures of food/fluids; popsicles are advised for moisture
  - **N&V:** Antiemetics as prescribed, hold foods and oral fluid 4-6hr before chemotherapy, frequent small bland meals, nutritional supplements
  - **Diarrhea:** Antidiarrheals as prescribed, monitor F&E, clear fluids, perineal care
  - **Anemia:** ↑Rest, monitor Hgb and Hct, give erythropoietin and transfusions if prescribed
  - **Neutropenia:** Monitor WBC, protect from infection (neutropenic precautions), give granulocyte colony-stimulating factor as prescribed
  - **Thrombocytopenia:** Monitor platelets, protect from injury, avoid injections or use smallest needle and apply pressure, use soft toothbrush, give platelets if prescribed
  - **Alopecia:** Emotional support, emphasize hair will grow back but may be different color/texture, encourage wig purchase and cut hair before chemo starts, wide-tooth comb to ↓trauma to hair, mild shampoo, avoid hair dryers and curling irons

Breast Cancer

Etiology and Pathophysiology
- Development of malignant cells due to hormonal, genetic and/or environmental factors
- Localized or invasive
- May affect lobules (**lobular carcinoma**) or ducts (**ductal carcinoma**)
- Ductal carcinoma associated with an itchy, scaly nipple lesion (**Paget's disease**)
- Stage 0 (in situ), Stage 1 (tumor <2cm), Stage 2 (tumor 2-5cm), Stage 3 (tumor >5cm), Stage 4 (metastasis)

Risk Factors
- ↑Age, female gender, family history, BRCA-1 and -2 genes
- No or late 1st pregnancy, estrogen replacement, early menarche, late menopause
- Alcohol, obesity, cancer in other breast

Signs and Symptoms
- Hard, nontender mass; often superior lateral breast
- May attach to underlying tissue (fixed)
- Recent inversion or flattening of nipple
- Unilateral venous prominence
- Orange peel appearance of breast tissue (**peau d' orange**)
- Enlarged axillary nodes
- Diagnostic tests: Mammogram, sonogram, MRI, tumor biopsy, sentinel node biopsy (identifies primary axillary node for breast drainage and need for standard vs. invasive axillary node dissection), estrogen receptor and progesterone receptor assays determine tumor's sensitivity to hormones, scans and tumor markers (Ca 15–3, Ca 125, carcinoembryonic antigen) determine progression

Treatment
- Based on stage
- Surgery (lumpectomy, mastectomy, nodal dissection)
- Reconstruction surgery involves progressive addition of saline into temporary implants to expand tissue before insertion of final implants; patient's own muscle flaps from abdomen or back are used to simulate breast tissue; tissue from inner thigh or labia is used to create nipple; tattoo to simulate areola
- Radiation, chemotherapy, hormonal therapy, bone marrow transplantation

(Continued text on following page)

Nursing

Monitor S&S
- Teach monthly breast self-examination (BSE):
  - Systematic light, medium, and deep palpation with finger pads over breasts and axilla once a month
  - 5–7 days after start of menses in premenopausal women and same day every month in postmenopausal women
  - Inspect for symmetry, dimpling, or nipple inversion
- Teach postmastectomy exercises (wall climbing) to ↑ muscle strength, ↓contractures, ↑risk of lymphedema
- Care related to chemotherapy see Pharmacology TAB 7
- Radiation: Manage fatigue, protect skin from irritation and sun, no ointments, lotions, or powders
- Postoperative:
  - Provide for pain management
  - Maintain self-suction drainage device to ↓edema
  - Protect extremity: No BPs or IVs, wear gloves for gardening, avoid lifting or carrying heavy items, use electric razor for axillary hair
- Provide support of patient and partner; refer to Reach to Recovery

Cervical Cancer

Etiology and Pathophysiology
- 90% from squamous cells; 10% from adenocarcinoma
- ↑Cure rate if diagnosed in situ

Risk Factors
- 30–45yr, human papillomavirus, initial sexual activity at young age, multiple sex partners, HIV

Signs and Symptoms
- Early: Watery vaginal secretion initially → foul-smelling discharge; bleeding between menses (**metrorrhagia**) or after intercourse
- Late: Back and leg pain, dysuria, rectal bleeding, anemia, ↑weight, abnormal Pap smear

Treatment
- Based on stage
- Cryotherapy or laser therapy, removal of part of cervix that maintains reproductive function (**conization**), hysterectomy, loop electrocautery excision procedure
- External radiation, intracavity radiation (**brachytherapy**)

Nursing
- Pregnant nurse must not care for patient receiving internal radiation
- **Internal radiation:**
  - Consider time/distance/shielding
  - Supine position, indwelling catheter
  - ↓Residue diet and antidiarrheals to ↓risk of dislodging insert
  - Organize care to ↓time in room
  - Provide emotional support
- **Postoperative:** Assess for bleeding and infection, pain management, incentive spirometry, DVT prevention

Ovarian Cancer

Etiology and Pathophysiology
- 90% epithelial
- Lower incidence than other GYN cancers but ↑mortality since most metastasize before diagnosis

Risk Factors
- Breast cancer, BRCA-1 and -2 genes, Caucasians (lowest for Asians)
- Industrialization, ↑fat diet, oral contraceptives, nulliparity, multipara

Signs and Symptoms
- May be asymptomatic until advanced
- ↑Abdominal girth 2° tumor or ascites
- Constipation, ↓weight, flatulence
- Anemia, enlarged ovary, urinary frequency, leg or pelvic pain
- ↑Ca-125 tumor antigen
- Tumor seen on transvaginal ultrasound

Treatment
- Total abdominal hysterectomy (uterus, ovaries, fallopian tubes, omentum)
- Chemotherapy with cyclophosphamide, doxorubicin, paclitaxel, cisplatin
- Ca-125 levels to assess progress
- Paracentesis or thoracentesis for palliation

Nursing
- Provide emotional support
- **Postoperative:**
  - Assess for bleeding and infection
  - Provide for pain management
  - Encourage incentive spirometry
  - Implement DVT prevention
  - Provide care related to side effects of chemotherapy (see Pharmacology TAB)

Infectious Diseases

Lyme Disease and Tetanus

	Lyme Disease	Tetanus (Lockjaw)
Etiology and Pathophysiology	*Borrelia burgdorferi:* Spirochete; infected deer or mouse → tick → human through tick's bite; 3–30 day incubation	*Clostridium tetani:* Anaerobic bacillus; enters puncture wound resulting in bacterial toxins affecting nervous system → muscle spasms; 3–21 day incubation
Risk factors	Northeastern U.S., wooded areas	No tetanus toxoid to produce active immunity
S&S	Early: Bull's-eye rash; Later: Arthritis, Bell's palsy, meningitis, carditis, dementia, and paralysis	Spasms of voluntary muscles causing pain, abnormal postures and facial expressions; Respiratory spasms and failure
Treatment	Amoxicillin, doxycycline, ceftriaxone	Tetanus immune globulin, supportive care
Nursing	Provide supportive care; Teach: Complete antibiotic therapy; wear long, light-color clothes to see tick; avoid tall grass; use repellent; inspect skin; use tweezers to remove tick	Maintain airway; Immune globulin for brief passive immunity; Wound care; Teach need for tetanus toxoid boosters q10yr for active immunity

Rabies and West Nile Virus

	Rabies	West Nile Virus (WNV)
Etiology and Pathophysiology	*Rhabdovirus:* Virus enters via bite from contaminated animal; infects tissue and CNS causing nerve destruction 4–21 day incubation	*Flavivirus:* Virus; infected birds → mosquitoes → human host 5–15 day incubation Risk of encephalitis or meningitis in infants, immunocompromised and older adults
Risk factors	Infected animal contact (bat, dog)	Eastern U.S., hot humid conditions
S&S	Irritability, thirst, throat spasms, ↑frothy salivation, dyspnea, paresthesia, seizures Death if untreated	Most symptom-free Headache, malaise, rash, lymphadenopathy, + IgM antibody to WNV Neurological S&S
Treatment	Rabies vaccine Immune globulin Anticonvulsants prn	No specific treatment Supportive care only
Nursing	Maintain airway Provide wound care Teach need to complete 6 doses of vaccine for active immunity	Provide supportive care Teach to eliminate standing water where mosquitoes breed; use repellent; wear long sleeves, pants, and gloves to touch dead bird

Common Therapeutic Drug Classes

Antacids: ↓Gastric Acidity, Protect Stomach Mucosa, and ↓Epigastric Pain

Mechanism of Action	Examples	Nontherapeutic Effects
Antacids: Bind with excess acid	magnesium/aluminum hydroxide (Maalox, Mylanta) aluminum hydroxide (Amphojel)	Aluminum salts ↑stool transit causing constipation and hypophosphatemia Magnesium salts ↑ peristalsis causing diarrhea and hypermagnesemia

Nursing Implications
- Many antacids contain Na, which should be avoided on ↑Na diets
- Shake suspensions well; give 60mL water to ↓ passage to stomach
- Encourage foods high in calcium and iron; avoid foods that ↑GI distress
- Caution about overuse, which may cause rebound hyperacidity
- Assess for presence/extent/relief of epigastric/abdominal pain
- Assess emesis and stool for frank/occult blood
- Teach need to see MD if symptoms do not resolve in 2wk
- Monitor serum calcium and phosphate levels with chronic use

Antidiarrheals: ↓Diarrhea; ↑ Production of Formed Stool

Mechanism of Action	Examples	Nontherapeutic Effects
Motility suppressants: ↑Motility so water is absorbed by large intestine	diphenoxylate HCI (Lomotil) loperamide (Imodium)	Tachycardia, respiratory depression, ileus, urinary retention, sedation, dry mouth
Enteric bacteria replacements: ↑Patho- genic bacterial growth	lactobacillus acidophilus (Bacid)	Abdominal cramps and ↓Flatulence

Nursing Implications
- Assess for frequency of bowel movements and color, characteristics of stool; assess bowel sounds for ↓in hyperactivity
- Monitor for F&E imbalances, particularly dehydration

Antibiotics/Anti-infectives: Destroy or ↓Growth of Susceptible Microorganisms

Mechanism of Action	Examples	Nontherapeutic Effects
Aminoglycosides: ↓Protein synthesis	gentamicin (Garamycin)	N&V, hypersensitivity reactions (rash, anaphylaxis)
Cephalosporins: Bind to cell wall causing cell death	cefazolin (Ancef) cephalexin (Keflex)	
Fluoroquinolones: ↓DNA synthesis	ciprofloxacin (Cipro) levofloxacin (Levaquin)	
Macrolides: ↓Protein synthesis	azithromycin (Zithromax) clarithromycin (Biaxin)	
Penicillins: Bind to cell wall → cell death	amoxicillin (Amoxil) penicillin V (Veetids, Pen-Vee)	
Sulfonamides: ↓Protein synthesis	doxycycline (Vibramycin)	
Anti-infective: ↓Protein and DNA synthesis; bactericidal, trichomonacidal, and amebicidal	metronidazole (Flagyl)	

Nursing Implications

- Ensure C&S before starting med; assess S&S of hepatotoxicity, nephrotoxicity, hyperglycemia, and drug interactions associated with some fluoroquinolones
- Assess S&S of infection
- Assess for signs of superinfection: Furry overgrowth on tongue, vaginal discharge, foul-smelling stools
- Administer evenly spaced doses to maintain blood levels
- Teach regimen should be completed to prevent resistance
- Do not crush/chew extended-release tablets
- Obtain blood specimen 1-3hr after a dose to measure highest level of med (peak) and 30-60min before next dose to measure lowest serum level of med (trough)

Anticoagulants: Interfere With Normal Coagulation to ↑ Thrombus Formation/Extension

Mechanism of Action	Examples	Nontherapeutic Effects
Thrombin inhibitors: Conversion of prothrombin to thrombin, thus ↓conversion of fibrinogen to fibrin	heparin lepirudin (Refludan)	Excessive bleeding (bruising), hematuria, epistaxis, bleeding gums), melena, ↑Hgb/Hct, anemia, thrombocytopenia
Low molecular weight heparins: Block coagulation factor Xa	dalteparin (Fragmin) enoxaparin (Lovenox)	
Clotting factor inhibitors: Interfere with hepatic synthesis of vitamin K and dependent clotting factors	warfarin (Coumadin)	
Platelet inhibitors: ↑Platelet aggregation	clopidogrel (Plavix) ticlopidine (Ticlid) aspirin	

Nursing Implications

- Discontinue anticoagulants before invasive procedures; notify MD if bleeding occurs; prepare to administer antidote: protamine sulfate for heparin and vitamin K for warfarin. Use medical alert card/jewelry.
- Assess for bleeding; monitor coagulation studies and platelet count; use electric razor, soft toothbrush
- Teach to avoid OTC medications, especially aspirin/NSAIDs
- Avoid alcohol and foods ↑ in vitamin K as they ↓med effectiveness
- **Thrombin inhibitors:** Monitor partial thromboplastin time (PTT-therapeutic level: 1.5–2.5 times control); half-life of heparin is 1–2hr
- **Low molecular weight heparins:** Do not use with another heparin product; if excessive bruising occurs, ice cube massage site before injection
- **Clotting factor inhibitors:** Monitor prothrombin time (PT-therapeutic level: 1.3–2.0 times control) or International Normalized Ratio (INR-therapeutic level: 2–4.5 times control)

210

Antiemetics: ↓N&V; Prevent and ↓Motion Sickness

Mechanism of Action	Examples	Nontherapeutic Effects
Phenothiazines: ↓Chemoreceptor trigger zone in CNS	prochlorperazine (Compazine) promethazine (Phenergan)	Confusion, photosensitivity, sedation, constipation, dry mouth, extrapyramidal reactions
5 HT₃ antagonists: Block serotonin at receptor sites in vagal nerve terminals and chemoreceptor trigger zone in CNS	ondansetron (Zofran)	Headache, dizziness, constipation, diarrhea
Anticholinergics: Correct imbalance of acetylcholine and norepinephrine in CNS that causes motion sickness	scopolamine (Transderm Scop) trimethobenzamide (Tigan)	Drowsiness; scopolamine: urinary hesitancy, blurred vision, dry mouth, tachycardia; Tigan suppository: ↓BP and local irritation
Nonphenothiazines: Block chemoreceptor trigger zone in CNS; ↑GI motility and ↑gastric emptying	metoclopramide (Reglan)	Extrapyramidal reactions, restlessness, drowsiness, anxiety, depression

Nursing Implications

- Administer 30-60min before chemotherapy or activity that causes motion sickness
- Monitor VS, presence/extent/relief of N&V, abdominal distention
- Ensure safety because of CNS depression; avoid alcohol and other CNS depressants
- Monitor for **extrapyramidal reactions**: involuntary movements, grimacing, rigidity, shuffling walk, trembling
- Phenothiazines: Encourage sunscreen/protective clothing, assess for **neuroleptic malignant syndrome**: Hyperthermia, diaphoresis, unstable BP, dyspnea, stupor, muscle rigidity, urinary incontinence

Antifungals: ↓Fungal Growth		
Mechanism of Action	**Examples**	**Nontherapeutic Effects**
Systemic: Impair fungal plasma membrane	clotrimazole (Mycelex) fluconazole (Diflucan) nystatin (Mycostatin)	Renal, liver, and ototoxicity, teratogenic, F&E imbalance, N&V, diarrhea, rash, fever
Topical: Disrupt fungal cell wall and metabolism	clotrimazole (Lotrimin), ketoconazole (Nizoral) nystatin (Mycostatin) amphotericin B	Burning, irritation

Nursing Implications

- **Systemic:** Monitor for nephrotoxicity, hepatotoxicity, ototoxicity
- Complete entire regimen; prevent pregnancy; monitor for hypoglycemia in pt with DM
- **Topical:** Monitor for irritation; clean skin with tepid water before application
- Teach difference between "swish and swallow" and "swish and spit"
- Teach how to use/insert med and to abstain from intercourse

Antiparasitics: Cause Parasite Death		
Mechanism of Action	**Examples**	**Nontherapeutic Effects**
Parasiticidal: Directly absorbed into parasites and eggs (for scabies and lice)	lindane (Kwell)	CNS toxicity and seizures
	permethrin (Nix)	Pruritus, tingling
Anthelmintic: Prevents worm growth and reproduction (for pinworms)	mebendazole (Vermox)	Hypersensitivity (rash, anaphylaxis) abdominal pain

Nursing Implications

- Wash bedding, clothes, etc., in hot water and dryer; vacuum carpets/furniture; seal nonwashables in plastic bags for 2wk; treat all family members
- **Pediculosis/scabies:** Use gown, gloves, hair cap when giving care; scrub body with soap and water, dry, apply med; avoid wounds, mucous membranes, face, eyes
- **Pinworms:** Obtain specimen via cellophane tape test in AM; monitor perianal condition and for GI distress
- Teach handwashing before meals and after toileting
- **Head lice:** Shampoo for 5min; use fine-tooth comb to remove eggs

Analgesics, Antipyretics, Nonsteroidal Anti-inflammatory Drugs (NSAIDs): ↓Synthesis of Prostaglandins, Which ↓Pain, Fever, and Inflammation

Mechanism of Action	Examples	Nontherapeutic Effects
Analgesic only: Inhibits prostaglandins involved in pain and fever	acetaminophen (Tylenol)	Hepatic toxicity
Non-salicylate NSAID: Inhibits prostaglandins involved in inflammation, pain, and fever	ibuprofen (Advil, Motrin) naproxen (Aleve, Naprosyn)	Rash, tinnitus, flulike syndrome
Salicylates NSAID: Inhibits prostaglandins involved in inflammation, pain, and fever	acetyl salicylic acid (aspirin, Ecotrin)	Agitation, hyperventilation, lethargy, confusion, diarrhea; **toxicity:** diaphoresis, tinnitus (8th cranial nerve damage)

Nursing Implications

- To avoid toxicity, do not exceed recommended 24hr dose; withhold 1wk before invasive procedures because of ↓platelet aggregation and risk of bleeding; salicylates contraindicated in pregnancy, lactation, and children <2yr (associated with Reye syndrome)
- Give with 8oz water, sit up 15-30min after ingestion, give with food except for naproxen and ibuprofen
- Monitor for NSAID side effects: headache, drowsiness, dizziness, photosensitivity
- Monitor for GI bleeding (anemia, melena)
- Avoid alcohol and OTC drugs with analgesic, antipyretic properties
- D/C drug and notify MD of serious side effects
- **Acetaminophen:** Do not exceed >4g per 24hr period (↓hepatotoxicity)
- **Salicylates:** Monitor serum salicylate levels

Antihistamines: ↓Symptoms Associated With Allergy and Motion Sickness

Mechanism of Action	Examples	Nontherapeutic Effects
Antihistamines: Blocks histamine, which ↓allergic response and motion sickness	diphenhydramine (Benadryl) loratidine (Claritin)	Dry eyes and mouth, constipation, blurred vision, sedation

(Continued text on following page)

Antihypertensives (Also See Diuretics): ↑BP

Mechanism of Action	Examples	Nontherapeutic Effects
Angiotensin antago- nists (ACE inhibitors): ↑Release of aldoster- one → ↓ excretion of sodium and water	enalapril maleate (Vasotec) fosinopril (Monopril) lisinopril (Prinivil, Zestril) ramipril (Altace)	Teratogenic, cough, taste disturbances, proteinuria, agranulocytosis, angioedema, neutropenia
Calcium channel blockers: ↑Relaxation and dilation of coronary smooth muscle of coronary arteries and arterioles	amlodipine (Norvasc) diltiazem HCl (Cardizem) nifedipine (Procardia) verapamil (Calan)	Flushing, peripheral edema; avoid use of calcium containing antacids or calcium supplements Cardizem, Calan: bradycardia
Angiotensin II receptor antagonists: ↑↑Vasoconstriction and ↑ release of aldosterone	irbesartan (Avapro) losartan (Cozaar) valsartan (Diovan)	Teratogenic, nephrotoxic; may cause angioedema; dyspnea, facial swelling
Beta blockers (selective): Block stimulation of beta1 (myocardial) adrenergic receptors	metoprolol (Lopressor) metoprolol tartrate (Toprol XL)	Fatigue, weakness, impotence, bradycardia, pulmonary edema; may ↑blood glucose of pts with DM
Beta blockers (nonselec- tive): Block stimulation of beta1 (myocardial) and beta2 (pulmonary, vascular, uterine) adrenergic receptors	carvedilol (Coreg) labetalol (Normodyne) propranolol (Inderal)	Fatigue, weakness, pulmonary edema; bradycardia, impotence
Centrally acting antiadre- nergics: Stimulate CNS alpha2 adrenergic re- ceptors ↑ sympa- thetic outflow	methyldopa (Aldomet)	Dizziness, weakness, dry mouth, constipation; may cause impotence

Nursing Implications

- Contraindicated with narrow-angle glaucoma; use caution with opioids—may cause paradoxic effect
- Exerts antiemetic, anticholinergic; CNS depressant effects; assess older adults for confusion
- May be used to promote sleep; assess older adults for falls risk
- Caution pt to avoid hazardous activities; monitor level of sedation
- Administer with food/fluid to ↓GI irritation
- Administer 1hr before activity for motion sickness prophylaxis
- Suggest use of gum/hard candy to ↑ salivation and ↓dry mouth
- Teach to wear clothing and sunscreen

Nursing Implications

- Abrupt withdrawal may cause life-threatening ↑BP or dysrhythmias; notify MD of dyspnea, severe dizziness, P is ↑, ↓, or irregular, persistent headache or ↑ or ↓ BP
- Monitor BP and P for rate, rhythm, and volume before administration and routinely; teach to monitor P daily and BP twice weekly; hold drug if P is below parameter set by MD (e.g., 50 beats/min)
- Assess for ↑fluid volume: ↑BP, intake ↑ than output, ↑wt, edema, breath sounds for crackles, bounding P, distended neck veins
- Monitor when using IV route: VS q 5-15min, ECG, pulmonary capillary wedge pressure, CVP
- Teach to take at same time each day, not to crush/break/chew extended-release tabs
- Avoid OTC meds, particularly cold remedies
- Ensure safety related to orthostatic hypotension, avoidance of hazardous activities
- Encourage actions to ↓BP (↓wt, ↓Na diet, exercise, avoid smoking and alcohol intake, stress management)
- Assess for headache, hypotension, dizziness, nausea, dysrhythmias, ↑sensitivity to cold; may cause impotence

Antilipidemics (Lipid Lowering): ↓Serum LDL, Triglycerides, and Total Cholesterol Levels; ↑HDL Levels

Mechanism of Action	Examples	Nontherapeutic Effects
HMG-CoA reductase inhibitors: Inhibit the enzyme (HMG-CoA)—a catalyst in synthesis of cholesterol	atorvastatin (Lipitor), rosuvastatin (Crestor), simvastatin (Zocor)	N&V, abdominal cramps, diarrhea, constipation, muscle soreness, hepatotoxicity, ↓absorption of fat-soluble vitamins
Bile acid sequestrants: Bind cholesterol in GI tract	cholestyramine (Questran)	
Fibrates: Inhibit peripheral lipolysis; ↓triglyceride production and synthesis	fenofibrate (Tricor), gemfibrozil (Lopid)	
Cholesterol absorption inhibitors: Inhibit absorption of cholesterol in small intestine	ezetimibe (Zetia)	

(Continued text on following page)

Mechanism of Action	Examples	Nontherapeutic Effects
Water-soluble vitamins: Inhibit release of free fatty acids from adipose tissue; ↑hepatic lipo-protein synthesis	niacin	

Nursing Implications

- Call MD for muscle pain, tenderness, or weakness with fever or malaise; **fibrates may ↑effect of warfarin**
- Encourage ↓cholesterol, ↓fat, ↑fiber, and fish high in omega-3 fatty acids (2-3 times a wk)
- Monitor serum cholesterol/triglycerides, Hgb, RBC, liver function studies
- Exchange vegetable oils with polyunsaturated fatty acids (PUFA) to those with monounsaturated fatty acids (MUFA)
- **HMG-CoA reductase inhibitors:** Take at hs; avoid grapefruit juice, which ↑risk of toxicity
- **Bile acid sequestrants:** Take ac with 8oz water; contraindicated for pts with phenylketonuria (PKU)
- **Fibrates:** May ↑anticoagulant effect of warfarin
- **Cholesterol absorption inhibitors:** Not advised during pregnancy and lactation
- **Water-soluble vitamins:** Transient sensation of warmth may occur; ensure safety if orthostatic hypotension present

Antineoplastics and Related Medications: Destroy or ↑Growth of Neoplastic Cells to Cure, Control, and/or Palliate

Mechanism of Action	Examples	Nontherapeutic Effects
Alkylating agents: ↑DNA synthesis preventing replication	carboplatin (Paraplatin) cisplatin (Platinol) cyclophosphamide (Cytoxan)	Myelosuppression, hypersensitivity, renal, GI, 2nd malignancies, skin problems **cisplatin:** nephrotoxic, ototoxic, neuropathies, vesicant **cyclophosphamide:** hemorrhagic cystitis
Antiandrogens: Block testosterone effect at cellular level	bicalutamide (Casodex) flutamide (Eulexin)	Hot flashes, gynecomastia, ↑libido

Antineoplastics and Related Medications: Destroy or ↓Growth of Neoplastic Cells to Cure, Control, and/or Palliate *(Continued)*		
Mechanism of Action	**Examples**	**Nontherapeutic Effects**
Antiangiogenic agents: ↓New blood vessel formation in tumors	bevacizumab (Avastin) thalidomide (Thalomid)	**bevacizumab:** Hypersensitivity, GI perforation, HTN, bleeding, ↓wound healing, arterial thromboembolic events **thalidomide:** birth defects, sedation, neuropathy, orthostatic hypotension, edema, ↓WBC
Antiestrogens: Compete for estrogen-binding sites in tissue	tamoxifen (Nolvadex)	Hot flashes, N&V, ↓libido, vaginal bleeding
Antimetabolites: Nolvadex ↓DNA synthesis and metabolism; cell-cycle S-phase specific	capecitabine (Xeloda) fluorouracil (5-FU) methotrexate (Mexate) gemcitabine (Gemzar)	Myelosuppression, GI and skin problems, alopecia
Antitumor antibiotics: ↓DNA synthesis; doxorubicin is cell-cycle S-phase specific	bleomycin (Blenoxane) doxorubicin (Adriamycin) doxorubicin hydrochloride liposome (Doxil)	Myelosuppression, alopecia, skin and GI problems; organ toxicity **bleomycin:** pulmonary toxicity **doxorubicin:** red urine, cardiotoxicity
Aromatase inhibitors: ↓Aromatase, which ↓estrogen level	anastrozole (Arimidex) letrozole (Femara)	Headache, weakness, hot flashes, musculoskeletal pain
Cytokines— hematopoietic growth factors: ↑Proliferation and function of hematopoietic cells	erythropoietin (Procrit, Epogen): ↑RBCs filgrastim (Neupogen) pegfilgrastim (Neulasta): ↑WBCs	Bone and injection site pain, N&V

(Continued text on following page)

MEDS

Mechanism of Action	Examples	Nontherapeutic Effects
Cytokines—immune stimulants: ↑Immune system; ↓tumor cell replication and growth	interferon alfa-2b (Intron-A)	Flulike symptoms, myelosuppression
Monoclonal antibodies: Bind to specific receptor sites to ↓cell proliferation	cetuximab (Erbitux): colorectal cancer rituximab (Rituxan): non-Hodgkin lymphoma trastuzumab (Herceptin): HER$_2$ sites in breast	Fever, N&V, headache, hypersensitivity **cetuximab:** Rash, interstitial lung disease **rituximab:** Tumor lysis syndrome, myelosuppression **trastuzumab:** cardiotoxicity, diarrhea
Plant alkaloids: ↓Cell replication, cell-cycle specific	docetaxel (Taxotere) paclitaxel (Taxol) topotecan (Hycamtin) vinblastine (Velban) vincristine (Oncovin)	Alopecia, myelosuppression, diarrhea, N&V, hypersensitivity, neurotoxicity, vesicant
Tyrosine kinase inhibitors (biological response modifiers): ↓Tumor growth; ↑cell death	erlotinib (Tarceva)	N&V, rash, photosensitivity
Combination therapy: Concurrent use of multiple drugs to destroy rapidly proliferating cells at different stages of replication; lower doses of each med ↓toxicity and tumor cell resistance	CMF: cyclophosphamide, methotrexate, fluorouracil CDV: cyclophosphamide, doxorubicin, vincristine	Myelosuppression, alopecia, skin and GI problems; organ toxicity **bleomycin:** pulmonary toxicity **doxorubicin:** red urine, cardiotoxicity

Nursing Care for Nontherapeutic Effects of Antineoplastic Meds

- **Call MD or NP if infection, bleeding, F&E imbalances, tumor lysis syndrome, nephrotoxicity, hepatotoxicity, or cardiotoxicity occur.**
- **Anorexia**
  - Calorie count
  - ↑Protein and calories
  - Small frequent meals; support food preferences
  - Supplements between meals
- **Nausea and vomiting**
  - Assess for I&O and F&E imbalances
  - Prevent aspiration
  - Provide adequate hydration
  - Parenteral antiemetic as ordered (30-45min before and for 24hr after caustic med)
- **Inflammation of oral mucosa (stomatitis)**
  - Assess mucous membranes, gag reflex, and ability to chew or swallow
  - Avoid hot and spicy foods and fluids
  - Puree/fluid diet as ordered
  - Rinse mouth with normal saline q2hr
  - Sponge toothbrush, avoid mouthwash, remove dentures except when eating
  - Topical antiseptics (swish and spit, or swallow)
- **Rectal sores or bleeding**
  - Assess for occult or frank blood in stool
  - Apply topical ointments/warm compresses as ordered
  - Avoid suppositories and rectal temps
- **Alopecia**
  - Assess self-esteem
  - Use mild shampoo
  - Use wide-tooth comb; minimize combing
  - Wear hat in the sun; purchase wig before hair loss
- **Diarrhea**
  - Assess perianal skin; S&S of F&E imbalance
  - Apply barrier ointment
- **Fatigue**
  - Assess activity tolerance
  - Organize activities to provide uninterrupted rest
  - Balance activity/rest
  - Help delegate responsibilities to conserve energy

(Continued text on following page)

■ **Low platelets (thrombocytopenia)**
■ Assess for S&S of bleeding: ecchymosis, petechiae, hematuria, melena, hematemesis, hemoptysis, bleeding from gums or venipuncture sites, ↓platelets, ↓Hct, ↓Hgb
■ Avoid rectal temps
■ Use electric razor, emery board for nail care
■ Use smallest gauge needle for injections
■ Compress venipuncture site for 5–10min
■ Avoid aspirin, NSAIDs, and alcohol
■ Give platelets as ordered

■ **Low leukocytes (↓WBCs, neutropenia)**
■ Monitor WBC count
■ Administer filgrastim (Neupogen) to ↑ WBCs
■ Assess for S&S of infection (↑T, chills, diaphoresis)
■ Teach pt to avoid people with infections
■ Obtain specimen for C&S before antibiotic if necessary
■ Provide care for sites of microorganism growth (IV and catheter sites, wounds, skin folds, perineum, oral cavity)
■ When WBC < 1,000/mm3 provide a private room and eliminate fresh fruits, vegetables, and flowers/potted plants

■ **Low erythrocytes (↓RBCs)**
■ Monitor RBCs, Hgb, and Hct
■ Administer epoetin (Epogen) to ↑RBC
■ Assess for tachycardia, pallor, fatigue
■ Administer blood products (PRBCs)

■ **Nephrotoxicity**
■ Monitor BUN, creatinine, creatinine clearance, and F&E
■ Give 2-3L of fluid daily
■ Administer allopurinol (Zyloprim) as ordered to prevent uric acid crystals
■ Assess for S&S of gout

■ **Cardiotoxicity**
■ Assess for dyspnea, crackles, ↑RR
■ Assess for peripheral edema
■ Assess for tachycardia, dysrhythmias
■ Monitor daily for weight gain

■ **Hepatotoxicity**
■ Assess for N&V, malaise, bruising/bleeding, jaundice
■ Monitor liver function tests

- **Tissue necrosis from extravasation of a vesicant**
  - Monitor for infiltration or inflammation
  - D/C and restart in another vein if needed
  - Elevate extremity for 24hr
  - Ensure IV is in vein and patent
  - Document event and notify MD or NP
  - Apply ice or warm compresses as per protocol
- **Tumor lysis syndrome**
  - Destroyed tumor cells release excessive intracellular metabolites causing hyperkalemia, hypocalcemia, hyperphosphatemia, and hyperuricemia
  - Assess for F&E imbalances
  - Administer therapy as ordered (IV fluids, Kayexalate, Zyloprim, phosphate-binding gels)

Antituberculars: ↓Cough, ↓Sputum, ↓Fever, ↓Night Sweats; and produce negative culture for *M. tuberculosis*

Mechanism of Action	Nontherapeutic Effects
isoniazid (INH): ↓Mycobacterial cell wall synthesis and interferes with metabolism	Peripheral neuropathy (numbness, tingling, paresthesia), hepatotoxicity (jaundice, N&V, anorexia, amber urine, weakness, fatigue)
rifampin: ↓Mycobacterial RNA synthesis	Thrombocytopenia; hepatotoxicity; red/orange urine, other body fluids; N&V; abdominal pain; flatulence; diarrhea
ethambutol: ↓Mycobacterial RNA synthesis	Optic neuritis (↓visual acuity, temporary loss of vision, constriction of visual field, red/green color blindness, photophobia, eye pain); rash
pyrazinamide (PZA): Causes cellular destruction	Hyperuricemia (pain in great toe and other joints); hepatotoxicity; skin rash; anorexia; N&V

Nursing Implications
- Assess VS: Rate, depth, characteristics; breath sounds; color/characteristics of sputum
- Monitor liver/renal function studies, CBC, serum uric acid, visual/auditory tests
- Obtain specimens for mycobacterial tests to detect possible resistance
- Encourage avoidance of alcohol to ↓hepatotoxicity
- **isoniazid** (INH): Avoid aluminum-containing antacids within 1hr of INH; administer pyridoxine (vitamin B_6) if ordered to ↓neuropathy
- **rifampin:** Take on empty stomach; teratogenic; ↓effectiveness of oral contraceptives
- **ethambutol:** Take with food; do not breastfeed; eye exams monthly
- **pyrazinamide** (PZA): ↑Fluid to 2-3L daily

Antiretrovirals: Treat HIV and AIDS; Prevent ↓Severity of Viral Infections

Mechanism of Action	Example
Nucleoside analog reverse transcriptase inhibitors (NRTIs): Damage HIV's DNA interfering with ability to control host DNA	FTC = emtricitabine (Emtriva) 3TC = lamivudine (Epivir) ZDV = zidovudine (AZT, Retrovir) ABC = abacavir (Ziagen)
Non-nucleoside reverse transcriptase inhibitors (NNRTIs): Prevent conversion of HIV RNA into HIV DNA	EFV = efavirenz (Sustiva) TDF = tenofovir (Viread)
Protease inhibitors: Inhibits HIV protease preventing virus maturation	RTV = ritonavir (Norvir) LPV/r = lopinavir/ritonavir (Kaletra)
Multiple drug regimens for naive pts: First time on highly active antiretroviral therapy (HAART) EFV + (3TC or FTC) + (ZDV or TDF); LPV/r + (3TC or FTC) + ZDV	**Atripla** (EFV + TDF + FTC) **Combivir** (AZT + 3TC) **Epzicom** (ABC + 3TC) **Kaletra** (LPV + RTV) **Trizivir** (AZT + 3TC + ABC) **Truvada** (FTC + TDF)

Nontherapeutic Effects

- Anorexia, N&V, diarrhea, headache, dizziness, vaginitis, moniliasis
- Additional effects depending on drug: Confusion, skin eruptions, allergic response, neuropathies, nephrotoxicity, blood dyscrasias, hepatotoxicity, CNS depression

Nursing Implications

- Explain that GI complaints and insomnia resolve after 3–4wk of treatment
- Encourage sexual abstinence or use of safer sex practices
- Encourage routine medical supervision; blood studies q2mo
- Refer to manufacturer's insert about need to take with or without food and what to do if a dose is missed
- Take meds exactly as prescribed; avoid OTC meds; compliance of 95% necessary to prevent resistance
- Assess for S&S of opportunistic infections
- Assess for S&S of nephrotoxicity, hepatotoxicity, and blood dyscrasias

Antivirals: Prevent or ↓Severity of Viral Infections and Symptoms (Not a Cure)

Mechanism of Action	Disease Treated
oseltamivir (Tamiflu): ↓Entry of virus into host	Influenza type A
acyclovir (Zovirax) **valacyclovir (Valtrex):** ↓Viral DNA synthesis	Herpes viruses: simplex, genitalis, zoster, varicella
ganciclovir (Cytovene): ↓Viral DNA synthesis	Cytomegalovirus

Nontherapeutic Effects

- Anorexia, N&V, diarrhea, headache, dizziness, vaginitis, moniliasis;
- Depending on drug: Confusion, skin eruptions, allergic response, neuropathies, nephrotoxicity, hepatotoxicity, blood dyscrasias, CNS depression

Nursing Implications

- Obtain C&S before starting therapy
- Take meds exactly as ordered to maintain therapeutic blood levels; avoid OTC medications
- Assess for S&S of nephrotoxicity, hepatotoxicity, and blood dyscrasias
- Assess for S&S of opportunistic infections
- **oseltamivir:** Begin treatment as soon as S&S appear, give at least 4hr before hs to ↓insomnia
- **acyclovir, valacyclovir:** Take for pain/pruritus, which usually occurs before eruptions; ↑fluids to 3L/d; herpes genitalis: ↑risk for cervical cancer, avoid sexual activity during exacerbations
- **ganciclovir:** Give with food; assess for neutropenia, thrombocytopenia, photosensitivity, ↓visual acuity; ensure regular ophthalmological exams; avoid pregnancy during and for 90 d after Tx (teratogenic); may cause infertility

Bronchodilators: Promote Bronchial Expansion, ↑Transfer of Gases, ↓Wheezing/Dyspnea

Mechanism of Action	Examples	Nontherapeutic Effects
Sympathomimetics (beta-adrenergic blocking agents): Relax bronchial smooth muscle, ↓spasms	albuterol (Proventil)	Headache, restlessness, tremor; paradoxical bronchospasm (wheezing, dyspnea, tightness in chest)

(Continued text on following page)

Mechanism of Action	Examples	Nontherapeutic Effects
Xanthines: Relax bronchial smooth muscle; ↑spasms	theophylline	↑P, BP; palpitations, dysrhythmias; dizziness, headache, restlessness; give with food; monitor serum theophylline level (therapeutic: 10-20mcg/mL)
Anticholinergics: ↓Action of acetyl-choline receptors in bronchial smooth muscle	ipratropium (Atrovent)	Dizziness, headache, nervousness; ↑BP, palpitations, blurred vision, urinary retention, dry mouth; encourage pt to void before taking; to ↓urinary retention; lozenges to ↓dry mouth
Leukotriene receptor antagonists: ↑Edema, bron-choconstriction; inflammation	montelukast (Singulair)	Headache, weakness, N&V; give on an empty stomach
Inhaled and nasal route steroids: ↓Local inflamma-tory response and edema, ↑airway diameter	budesonide (Pulmicort) fluticasone (Flovent)	Headache, oropharyngeal fungal infections, dysphonia, hoarseness **budesonide:** Flulike syndrome

Nursing Implications

- Wait 1–5min between inhaled drugs; use bronchodilator first
- Use spacer with MDI to limit large droplets; rinse mouth after use
- Obtain return demonstration of use of meter, inhaler, nebulizer
- Assess breaths sounds, extent of wheezing, color and characteristics of sputum
- Monitor respiratory rate, depth, characteristics; heart for ↑rate and dysrhythmias; ↑BP
- Encourage use of all meds because of variety of purposes
- Teach to avoid smoking and other respiratory irritants
- Encourage intake of 2-3L of fluid daily to maintain hydration
- Call MD if SOB is ↑ or is accompanied by diaphoresis, dizziness, palpitations, chest pain
- **Sympathomimetics:** Use cautiously for pts with cardiac problems; avoid use with tricyclic antidepressants or MAO inhibitors (may → hypertensive crisis or dysrhythmias)
- **Xanthines:** Use cautiously for pts with cardiac problems
- **Anticholinergics:** Contraindicated with glaucoma

Antisecretory Agents: ↓Gastric Acidity and Pain

Mechanism of Action	Examples	Nontherapeutic Effects
H₂ antagonists: ↓Histamine at H_2 receptors in parietal cells → ↓gastric secretions	famotidine (Pepcid) ranitidine (Zantac)	Blood dyscrasias (↓RBC, ↓WBC, ↓platelets) CNS disturbances (confusion, dizziness, drowsiness, headache) Dysrhythmias; nephrotoxicity hypersensitivity reactions
Proton pump inhibitors: ↓entry of hydrogen ions into gastric lumen	esomeprazole (Nexium), omeprazole (Prilosec), lansoprazole (Prevacid), pantoprazole (Protonix)	

Nursing Implications
- May ↑anticoagulant effect of warfarin; CNS disturbances often occur in older adults
- Administer 1-2hr before/after antacids; give po meds with meals
- Assess heart rate and rhythm, emesis/stool for frank/occult blood, CBC for blood dyscrasias
- **H₂ antagonists:** Smoking interferes with drug action; may cause diarrhea
- **Proton pump inhibitors:** Do not crush/chew capsule

Diuretics: ↑Urine Output, ↓Hypervolemia, ↓BP, ↓Peripheral Edema, ↓ICP, ↓Intraocular Pressure, ↓Seizures

Mechanism of Action	Examples	Nontherapeutic Effects
Thiazides/thiazide-like: ↓Sodium and chloride resorption in distal convoluted tubule and ↓chloride resorption in ascending loop of Henle	**thiazide:** Hydrochlorothiazide (HCTZ) **thiazide-like:** Metolazone (Zaroxolyn)	Dehydration, orthostatic hypotension, F&E imbalances ↓Potassium (except potassium-sparing drugs)
Loop: ↓Sodium and chloride resorption in ascending loop of Henle and distal renal tubule	bumetanide (Bumex) furosemide (Lasix)	↑Potassium (potassium-sparing drugs) ↓Sodium, ↓chloride, ↓magnesium, ↑calcium Pain in great toe and other joints

(Continued text on following page)

Mechanism of Action	Examples	Nontherapeutic Effects
Potassium-sparing: spironolactone: acts in distal tubule: ↓action of aldosterone, ↓sodium and potassium excretion; **triamterene:** ↑excretion of sodium and blocks potassium loss	spironolactone (Aldactone) triamterene (Dyrenium)	CNS complications: dizziness, drowsiness, lethargy, weakness, hearing loss Photosensitivity Pulmonary edema N&V ↓Serum glucose
Carbonic anhydrase inhibitors: ↓Carbonic anhy-drase in proximal renal tubule thereby ↑excretion of Na, K, bicarbonate, and water (**diuretic effect**); ↑aqueous humor, which ↑intraocular pressure (**ophthalmic effect**); ↓abnormal paroxysmal discharge in CNS neurons (**anticonvulsant effect**)	acetazolamide (Diamox)	

Nursing Implications

- Assess for F&E imbalances, particularly hypo- and hyperkalemia, which can cause dysrhythmias
- Give in AM to ↓disruption in sleep; monitor VS before administration; monitor for S&S of hypervolemia (↑BP, bounding pulse, output exceeds intake, ↑wt, extent of pitting edema, breath sounds for crackles); S&S of hypovolemia (↓BP, weak thready pulse, tenting of skin, dry sticky mucous membranes)
- Avoid sun to ↑photosensitivity (sunscreen, protective clothing)
- Take meds even if feeling better; meds control, not cure, hypertension
- Change position slowly to ↓orthostatic hypotension
- Encourage other interventions to ↓BP (↓wt, ↓Na diet, ↓smoking, ↑exercise, stress management)

Thrombolytic Agents: Dissolve Clots in Blood Vessels or Venous/Arterial Catheters		
Mechanism of Action	**Examples**	**Nontherapeutic Effects**
Thrombolytics: Activates conversion of plasminogen to plasmin, which breaks down clots	reteplase streptokinase urokinase	Bleeding: GI/GU, retroperitoneal, CNS; ecchymoses; reperfusion arrhythmias; rash; dyspnea; anaphylaxis **streptokinase:** Periorbital edema, allergic reactions, bronchospasm, pulmonary emboli

Nursing Implications

- Used to treat coronary artery thrombi, pulmonary emboli, acute ischemic brain attack, DVT, arterial thromboembolism, occluded central venous access devices. Administer within 6hr, preferably 3hr; ↑risk of bleeding in pts older than 75yr, ≤ 10 d postpartum, or receiving warfarin, aspirin, NSAIDs, heparin, and heparin-like agents
- **Contraindications:** History of brain attack, recent surgery/trauma, uncontrolled HTN, bleeding tendencies, intracranial neoplasm, AV malformation
- Follow manufacturer's directions for solution/drug compatibility and infusion rate; use IV controller/pump
- Assess VS and for bleeding q15min 1st hr, q15-30min next 8hr, and then q4hr; assess for coffee-ground emesis, tarry stool, occult blood, hematuria, epistaxis; ↓neurological status, sudden severe headache (cranial bleed); joint pain, back and leg pain (retroperitoneal bleed); abdominal pain, T 104°F (internal bleed); hold med and call MD immediately for S&S of bleeding
- Monitor Hgb, Hct, platelets, APPT, PT, TT, INR, bleeding time
- Have blood and the antidote (aminocaproic acid [Amicar]) available in case of hemorrhage

Hypoglycemics (Oral): Control Blood Glucose in Type 2 Diabetes

Mechanism of Action	Examples	Nontherapeutic Effects
Sulfonylureas: Stimulates beta cells to release insulin	glimepiride (Amaryl) glipizide (Glucotrol) glyburide (Micronase)	Hypoglycemia
Biguanides: ↑Sensitivity to insulin, ↑binding of insulin to its receptor	metformin (Glucophage)	Lactic acidosis (drowsiness, hyperventilation, myalgia and malaise), hypoglycemia
Meglitinides: ↑Release of insulin in pancreas	repaglinide (Prandin)	Hypoglycemia
Thiazolidinediones: ↓Insulin action in muscle and fat, ↑gluconeogenesis	pioglitazone (Actos) rosiglitazone (Avandia)	Upper respiratory tract infection; hypoglycemia does not occur

Nursing Implications

- Contraindicated in type 1 diabetes, uncontrolled infection, pregnancy, breastfeeding, and serious burns, trauma, and renal, hepatic, or endocrine disease
- Monitor for hypoglycemia, hyperglycemia, and hyperosmolar nonketotic coma
- Perform finger stick for serum glucose; ketones in urine if blood glucose is ≥300
- Teach to avoid alcohol because it may produce Antabuse-like reaction
- Do not crush sustained-release tablets; take 30min before meal or follow MD orders
- See hyper- and hypoglycemia and related nursing care (Medical Surgical Nursing Tab 6)
- **Thiazolidinediones:** Monitor liver function

Insulins: Time-Action Profile of Different Insulins				
Insulin Type	**Examples**	**Onset**	**Peak**	**Duration**
Rapid acting	Lispro (Humalog)	Rapid	30–60min	3–4hr
	NovoLog (Aspart)	Rapid	40–50min	4–6hr
Fast acting	Regular (Reg, R)	30–60min	2–4hr	5–7hr
	Regular IV	10–30min	15–30min	30–60min
Intermediate acting	NPH	1–4hr	6–12hr	18–28hr
Long acting	Lantus (Glargine)	1hr	Continuous	24hr
Combinations	NPH/Reg (70/30)	30min	4–8hr	24hr

Nursing Implications
- Only regular insulin can be given via IV
- Roll, do not shake vials of insulin
- Use calibrated insulin syringe to ensure accuracy

Procedure for Mixing Insulins

Proper techniques prevent NPH insulin from ↓purity of solution in the fast-acting Regular insulin vial

1. Use insulin syringe calibrated in units (0.3, 0.5, 1.0mL; 1/2, 5/8, 1.0in needle).
2. Draw up air equal to combined volume of both insulins.
3. Inject NPH vial with amount of air equal to ordered amount of NPH without dipping needle into solution. (Keep vial right side up.)
4. Inject remaining air into Reg insulin vial, invert vial, and draw up the ordered amount of Reg insulin; expel any air/bubbles.
5. Reinsert needle into NPH vial, invert vial, and withdraw ordered amount.

Laxatives and Cathartics: ↓Constipation; Evacuate Bowel for Diagnostic Tests or Surgery

Mechanism of Action	Examples	Nontherapeutic Effects
Bulk-forming: ↑Bulk stimulates peristalsis	methylcellulose (Citrucel) psyllium (Metamucil)	Cramps F&E imbalances Dependence
Stool softeners: Water and fat enters feces to soften and ↓drying of stool	docusate sodium (Colace)	
Stimulant/Irritants: Irritates ← rapid pro- pulsion of contents	bisacodyl (Dulcolax) cascara/senna (Senokot, Ex-Lax)	
Lubricants: Softens feces	mineral oil	
Saline osmotics: Draws water into intestinal lumen distending bowel stimulating peristalsis	magnesium salts (Milk of Magnesia) sodium phosphate (Fleet Phospho-Soda)	

Nursing Implications
- Contraindicated with N&V, abdominal pain, or signs of acute abdomen (may indicate bowel obstruction); do not use Na osmotic with older adults or children—may cause F&E imbalances
- Encourage ↑fluid intake, activity, dietary fiber; assess stool frequency, consistency
- Administer at bedtime
- **Bulk-forming:** Mix in 8oz of fluid and follow with 8oz fluid; may take ≥12hr to act
- **Stool softeners:** May take several days to act
- **Stimulant/Irritants:** Acts quickly; fluid may be passed with feces
- **Lubricants:** May ↓absorption of fat-soluble vitamins
- **Saline osmotics:** Rapid acting; may cause dehydration, hypernatremia, ↓absorption of fat-soluble vitamins

Opioid (Narcotic) Antagonists: Reverse Opiate Induced CNS Depression and ↓Respiratory Function

Mechanism of Action	Examples	Nontherapeutic Effects
Opioid antagonist: Displaces opioid at respiratory receptor sites via competitive antagonism	naloxone HCl (Narcan)	N&V, ↓↑BP, ventricular fibrillation

Nursing Implications

- Monitor VS, particularly respiratory rate and BP
- Monitor for opioid withdrawal (restlessness, ↑BP, ↑temp, abdominal cramps, N&V)

Opioid Analgesics: ↓Transmission of Pain Impulses; ↓Cough; ↓GI Motility to Treat Diarrhea

Mechanism of Action	Examples	Nontherapeutic Effects
Opioid analgesics: Combine with opioid receptors in CNS	codeine fentanyl (Duragesic): 72hr transdermal patch for chronic pain hydrocodone (Hycodan) hydromorphone (Dilaudid) methadone HCL (Dolophine) morphine (MS Contin, Roxanol): for intractable pain, MI, pulmonary edema oxycodone (OxyContin)	↓Respiratory rate, sedation, constipation, nausea, drowsiness, pruritus **fentanyl citrate:** Dry mouth, diaphoresis, weakness

Opioid/Nonopioid Analgesic Combinations:
propoxyphene napsylate and acetaminophen (Darvocet-N)
hydrocodone and acetaminophen (Vicodin)
oxycodone and acetaminophen (Percocet)
codeine phosphate and
acetaminophen
(Tylenol w/codeine 1, 2, 3, or 4)

(Continued text on following page)

Nursing Implications

- Monitor for respiratory depression; keep naloxone (Narcan) available for toxicity or overdose
- Give before pain is severe; regularly scheduled doses maintain therapeutic blood levels and ↑effectiveness
- Monitor pain, VS, respiratory depression (if R rate is ≤10/min, hold dose and call MD), hypotension, drowsiness, confusion, constipation, N&V, tolerance and dependence
- Give additional med for breakthrough pain; common with continuous infusion, sustained release med, or intractable pain
- Give combinations of opioids and analgesics cautiously; combinations ↑effectiveness (synergistic effect); may ↑toxicity
- Decrease slowly after chronic use to ↓S&S of withdrawal
- Encourage coughing and deep breathing every 2hr
- Limit constipation by ↑fluids, fiber, and activity; give stool softeners and laxatives if ordered
- Provide for safety; encourage avoidance of hazardous activities, change position slowly
- Use cautiously with ↑ICP (can mask S&S of increasing ICP)
- Teach how to self-administer med (IM, Sub-Q, sublingual, transdermal)

Obstetric Medications

Uterine relaxants: *magnesium sulfate, terbutaline sulfate (Brethine)*

- **Action:** ↓Uterine contractions
- **Contraindications:** HTN, DM, preeclampsia, <20th or >36th wk
- **Nursing:** Assess VS, BP, and S&S of preterm labor, tremor; provide emotional support

Uterine stimulants for labor: *oxytocin (Pitocin), misoprostol (Cytotec)*

- **Action:** ↑Uterine contractions to stimulate labor
- **Contraindications:** Cephalopelvic disproportion, malpresentation, fetal compromise, placenta previa, active genital herpes, uterine scar
- **Nursing:** Monitor fetal heart rate, uterine rupture (acute abd pain or rigidity, S&S of shock); D/C if contractions are <2min intervals or last ≥90min, then use left side-lying position, O_2. Prepare for cesarean birth

Uterine stimulants for postpartum bleeding: *prostaglandin (Hemabate), methylergonovine maleate (Methergine), nitroglycerine*

- **Action:** ↑Uterine tone to treat postpartum bleeding
- **Nursing:** Monitor bleeding; Hemabate: give antidiarrheal if ordered; Methergine: monitor for N&V

Uterine evacuation: *misoprostol (Cytotec), dinoprostone (Cervidil)*

- **Action:** Evacuate uterus for medical termination 12 to 28wk, after missed abortion or fetal demise
- **Nursing:** Insert following manufacturer's directions; monitor progress; Cervidil: monitor for ↑T; notify MD of chest tightness

Cervical softening agents: *dinoprostone (Prostin E2, Cervidil), Laminaria tent*

- **Action:** Cervical softening agents ↑effacement; follow with oxytocin to stimulate contractions
- **Nursing:** Insert gel, suppository, and Laminaria following manufacturer's directions; monitor fetal status, progress of labor; Cervidil: monitor for ↑T, notify MD of chest tightness (↑sensitivity)

RHo(D) Immune Globulin and Rho(D) Immune Globulin MICRO-Dose

- **Action:** Prevent isoimmunization in Rh-negative pt exposed to Rh-positive RBCs; protect against erythroblastosis fetalis in next Rh-positive pregnancy
- **Nursing:** Give within 72hr after birth/termination to eligible mother only; ensure vial is cross-matched to woman

Anticonvulsants: *Antihypertensives: magnesium sulfate, hydralazine (Apresoline), labetalol*

- **Action:** ↓Seizures in preeclampsia
- **Nursing:** Assess for ↓BP; ↓R; P for rate and rhythm; seizure precautions magnesium sulfate: assess pulmonary and neurological status; D/C for tightness in chest or absence of knee-jerk reflex; serum magnesium levels q6hr; warm flush is expected
- **Antihypertensives:** Monitor for ↓BP, ↑P, and F&E imbalance; maintain supine position during and 3hr after; assess newborn for hypotension, respiratory depression, and hyporeflexia

Glucocorticoids: *Betamethasone (Celestone), dexamethasone (Decadron)*

- **Action:** ↓Neonatal respiratory distress syndrome
- **Nursing:** Monitor for F&E imbalance, cerebral edema, adrenal insufficiency (↑wt, ↑BP, weakness, N&V, lethargy, confusion, restlessness); D/C slowly if used more than 1wk

Skeletal muscle relaxants: *central acting—cyclobenzaprine (Flexeril), diazepam (Valium); direct acting—dantrolene (Dantrium)*

- **Action:** ↓Muscle spasms; central acting: interfere with reflexes in upper CNS; direct acting: interfere with release of calcium from muscle tubules within skeletal muscles preventing contraction
- **Nursing:** Give with food/milk to ↓GI irritation; avoid hazardous activity until sedative response is known; avoid alcohol and other CNS depressants; ↓constipation: ↑fluids, ↑fiber, use stool softeners; monitor pain, muscle stiffness, and ROM routinely; encourage use of ordered rest, heat, physical therapy

Hormonal Disorders and Related Medications

Do not D/C any hormonal medications abruptly

Hyperthyroidism: Propylthiouracil (PTU), methimazole (Tapazole)

- **Action:** ↓Formation of thyroid hormone
- **Nontherapeutic effects:** Agranulocytosis (sore throat, fever, headache, malaise)
- **Nursing:** Report S&S of agranulocytosis to MD

Hyperthyroidism: Sodium iodine[131]

- **Action:** Destroy thyroid tissue
- **Nontherapeutic effects:** S&S of hypothyroidism: fatigue, lethargy, ↓wt, cold intolerance, constipation, dry skin
- **Nursing:** Use precautions for 6–8hr to 3–7 d as indicated; discard vomitus and excreta with multiple toilet flushes; avoid holding/hugging others or place in isolation 3–7 days as ordered

Hypothyroidism: Levothyroxine sodium (Synthroid, Levothroid)

- **Action:** Replace thyroid hormone
- **Nontherapeutic effects:** S&S of hyperthyroidism: ↑VS, irritability, insomnia, headache, dysrhythmias, ↓wt, diaphoresis, diarrhea, heat intolerance, fine hand tremor
- **Nursing:** Hold med and notify MD for resting P ≥100/min

Hyperparathyroidism: Calcitonin (Miacalcin)

- **Action:** ↑Renal excretion of calcium
- **Nontherapeutic effects:** Facial flushing; injection site reactions; hypersensitivity; hypocalcemia (muscle twitching, irritability, paresthesias, positive Chvostek's and Trousseau's signs)
- **Nursing:** Monitor for S&S of hypocalcemia

Diabetes insipidus: Vasopressin (Pitressin)

- **Action:** Antidiuretic
- **Nontherapeutic effects:** Water intoxication (confusion, drowsiness, headache, ↓wt, difficulty urinating, seizures)
- **Nursing:** Monitor S&S of water intoxication/dehydration; daily wt, I&O

Cushing syndrome: Aminoglutethimide (Cytadren), mitotane (Lysodren)

- **Action:** ↓Production of adrenal steroids
- **Nontherapeutic effects:** N&V, GI distress, depression, rash, vertigo, diplopia; many drug interactions
- **Nursing:** Monitor: VS, daily wt for adrenal insufficiency (fatigue, orthostatic hypotension, ↓wt, dehydration, GI distress, signs of shock); aminoglutethimide: used only for 3mo, monitor for hypothyroidism and CNS effects; mitotane: monitor for ↑hepatic function

235

Addison's disease: Hydrocortisone (Cortef), cortisone acetate (Cortone, Acetate)

- **Action:** Replacement therapy in adrenocortical insufficiency
- **Nontherapeutic effects:** Na and fluid retention, ↓wound healing, anaphylaxis, ↑wt, urinary frequency/urgency, vertigo, thrombophlebitis; and other CNS and cardiovascular problems
- **Nursing:** Generally larger dose in AM than afternoon as per orders (mimics circadian rhythm and ↓side effects); ↑dose needed when stressed; monitor VS, daily wt, F&E balance; protect from infection (meds mask infection), noise, light and extremes in environmental temperature

Addison's disease: Fludrocortisone (Florinef)

- **Action:** Mineralocorticoid replacement to manage Na loss and ↓BP
- **Nontherapeutic effects:** Heart failure, dizziness, headache, hypokalemia, adrenal suppression, ↑wt, edema
- **Nursing:** Monitor VS, fluid retention, electrolyte imbalances; ↓BP may indicate inadequate med dose

Excess growth hormone: Octreotide (Sandostatin)

- **Action:** ↓Growth hormone levels
- **Nontherapeutic effects:** Dizziness, drowsiness, orthostatic hypotension, visual disturbances, diarrhea
- **Nursing:** Assess VS, BP, S&S of gallbladder disease, diarrhea; store in refrigerator; give at room temp

Premature menopause; menopausal symptoms: estrogen, conjugated (Premarin)

- **Action:** Hormone replacement therapy (HRT)
- **Nontherapeutic effects:** Nausea, fluid retention, headache, breast tenderness, oily skin, amenorrhea, dysmenorrhea; contraindicated in pregnancy and breast cancer
- **Nursing:** Assess for S&S of cardiac disease, venous thrombosis, brain attack, pulmonary embolus; weigh daily and assess BP (can ↑ due to Na and water retention)
- May cause thromboembolic disorders; teach S&S of thrombophlebitis (extremity pain, swelling, tenderness), brain attack (headache, blurred vision), pulmonary embolus (chest pain, dyspnea, cough)

Erectile dysfunction: Sildenafil citrate (Viagra), tadalafil (Cialis)

- **Action:** ↑Strength and duration of erections
- **Nontherapeutic effects:** HTN, UTI, headache, insomnia, constipation, dry mouth
- **Nursing:** Teach: take 1hr before sex, only once daily, S&S of cardiac distress, drug interactions; call MD if erection lasts ≥4hr
- Fatal cardiovascular effects if used with nitrates (brain attack, MI)

Contraception: Oral monophasic, biphasic, triphasic formulations (combined estrogen/progestin in different doses and cycles)

- **Action:** ↑Ovulation by suppressing FSH and LH
- **Nontherapeutic effects:** Nausea, breakthrough bleeding, pigmentation of face, fluid retention, ↑BP, candidiasis, vaginal
- **Nursing:** Follow instructions for pill sequence and missed pills; assess for S&S of ectopic pregnancy; avoid breastfeeding
  Risk for thromboembolism; ↑pregnancy risk with use of antibiotics, phenobarbital, phenytoin, and rifampin; contraindications: ≥35yr old smoker, hx of thromboembolus; should have regular Pap smears, physicals, mammograms, and stop smoking

Contraception: Depot-medroxyprogesterone acetate (Depo-Provera); etonogestrel implant (Implanon)

- **Action:** ↓Sperm/ovum transport and ↓ovum implantation
- **Nontherapeutic effects:** Uterine bleeding, thromboembolus; Implanon: headache, ↑BP
- **Nursing:** Progesterone injection given 4 times a yr (Depo-Provera) or a 3yr subdermal implant (Implanon); Implanon: monitor site (midportion of upper arm); teach to replace within 3yr as effectiveness decreases
  Risk for thromboembolism; ↑pregnancy risk with use of antibiotics, phenobarbital, phenytoin, and rifampin; contraindications: ≥35yr old smoker, hx of thromboembolus; should have regular Pap smears, physicals, mammograms, and stop smoking

Emergency contraception: Levonorgestrel/ethinylestradiol (Preven), levonorgestrel (Plan-B)

- **Action:** ↓Implantation; 75% effective
- **Nontherapeutic effects:** Thromboembolism, nausea, abdominal pain, fatigue, headache, menstrual changes
- **Nursing:** Begin within 72hr after intercourse; contraception counseling
  Risk for thromboembolism; ↑pregnancy risk with use of antibiotics, phenobarbital, phenytoin, and rifampin; contraindications: ≥35yr old smoker, hx of thromboembolus; should have regular Pap smears, physicals, mammograms, and stop smoking

Prostate cancer: Leuprolide (Lupron)

- **Action:** Produces chemical castration; ↓testosterone
- **Nontherapeutic effects:** Bone pain, hot flashes, ↓libido, impotence
- **Nursing:** Monitor bone pain (will resolve with time), analgesics for pain

Prostate cancer: Flutamide (Eulexin), bicalutamide (Casodex)

- **Action:** Inhibits androgen uptake or binding
- **Nontherapeutic effects:** Hot flashes, ↓libido, impotence, breast pain and gynecomastia, diarrhea, hepatotoxicity
- **Nursing:** Assess for S&S of hepatotoxicity; notify MD

Psychotropic Medications
Anxiolytics, Sedatives and Hypnotics: ↓Anxiety; (Anxiolytic, Sedative); Induce Sleep (Hypnotic); Ease Alcohol Withdrawal

Mechanism of Action	Examples	Nontherapeutic Effects
Benzodiazepines: ↑Action of gamma-aminobutyric acid (GABA) inhibitory neurotransmitter	**Short acting:** alprazolam (Xanax) midazolam (Versed) **Medium acting:** lorazepam (Ativan) **Long acting:** chlordiazepoxide (Librium) clonazepam (Klonopin) diazepam (Valium)	↓Mental alertness, ↓BP, drowsiness, dizziness, headache, paradoxic reactions (euphoria, excitement)
Nonbarbiturates: All have CNS depressant effect, variable action depending on med	buspirone (BuSpar) diphenhydramine (Benadryl) hydroxyzine (Atarax, Vistaril) zolpidem (Ambien)	

Nursing Implications

- Barbiturates rarely used because of greater dependence and effectiveness of other agents
- Avoid alcohol/sedatives as they ↑drug effects
- Avoid caffeine, which ↓drug effects
- Avoid hazardous activities until tolerance develops
- Avoid concurrent use with herbal products (e.g., St. John's wort, kava, ginseng)
- Hold drug if systolic BP drops 20mm Hg on standing
- D/C gradually to prevent withdrawal; use longer than 2wk may lead to dependence
- **Buspirone:** Effect takes 3-6wk, which is longer than other anxiolytics

Antidepressants: Lift depressed Mood, ↓S&S of Panic Response, Narcolepsy, and S&S of Attention Deficit Disorder		
Mechanism of Action	**Examples**	**Nontherapeutic Effects**
Tricyclics (TCAs): ↓Reuptake of norepinephrine and serotonin into presynaptic nerve terminals	amitriptyline (Elavil) doxepin (Sinequan) nortriptyline (Pamelor)	Anticholinergic, ↓BP, and CNS stimulation effects
Selective serotonin reuptake inhibitors (SSRIs): ↓Reuptake of serotonin into presynaptic nerve terminals	citalopram (Celexa) fluoxetine (Prozac) paroxetine (Paxil) sertraline (Zoloft)	Sexual dysfunction, ↑appetite, anticholinergic and CNS stimulation/depression, hepatotoxicity, wt gain, photosensitivity
Monoamine oxidase inhibitors (MAOIs): ↓Breakdown of norepinephrine, dopamine, and serotonin in CNS neurons	phenelzine (Nardil)	Sexual dysfunction, rash, anticholinergic effects, and CNS stimulation/depression effects
Atypical new generation meds: ↑Effects of dopamine serotonin and/or norepinephrine at neural membranes	bupropion (Wellbutrin) mirtazapine (Remeron) venlafaxine (Effexor)	Drowsiness, dizziness, headache, insomnia, N&V, anticholinergic effects

Nursing Implications

- Assess for suicidal potential; particularly as mood lifts & physical/psychic energy increases
- Ensure a minimum of 2-6wk between concurrent use of TCAs, MAOIs or SSRIs to avoid serotonin syndrome; do not D/C drug abruptly
- Assess for anticholinergic and CNS effects
- Avoid prescription, OTC, or herbal products without supervision
- Take at hs if sedation occurs or in AM if insomnia occurs
- Avoid hazardous activities until sedative effect is known
- Change positions slowly to ↓orthostatic hypotension
- **Tricyclics (TCAs)**
  - Avoid giving with narrow-angle glaucoma or cardiac condition
  - Teach effect may take 2-6wk

- **SSRIs**
  - Teach that effect may take 5wk
  - Obtain baseline wt, monitor regularly
  - Teach exercise and ↓caloric intake to ↓wt gain and to wear protective clothing and sunscreen outdoors
- **MAOIs**
  - Avoid foods containing tyramine to prevent hypertensive crisis (aged cheese, beer, wine, chocolate, caffeine, licorice, bananas, raisins, pepperoni, salami, bologna, liver, sour cream, yogurt)
  - ↓BP may occur when given with an antihypertensive
  - Teach effect may take 4-8wk
- **New generation meds**
  - Give with food to ↓GI irritation; avoid chewing/crushing sustained-release capsules
  - Avoid alcohol during therapy because of potentiation
  - Monitor VS routinely for ↑BP and ↑P
  - Inform MD if pregnancy is planned
- **Wellbutrin and Remeron:** Assess for wt gain; space doses equally to ↓potential for seizures; seizure precautions

Antipsychotic Agents (Neuroleptics): ↓Agitated Behavior and Psychotic Symptoms (Positive and Negative Symptoms; Disorganized Thinking and Behavior)

Mechanism of Action	Examples	Nontherapeutic Effects
Typical (traditional) antipsychotics: For positive (type I) symptoms	chlorpromazine (Thorazine) haloperidol (Haldol) prochlorperazine (Compazine)	**Extrapyramidal tract side effects (EPS):** Dystonia (early in therapy), akathisia (most common), Parkinsonism, tardive dyskinesia (prolonged use)
Atypical antipsychotics: for negative (type II) symptoms	clozapine (Clozaril) olanzapine (Zyprexa) quetiapine (Seroquel) risperidone (Risperdal) ziprasidone (Geodon)	Sedation; ↓BP, sexual dysfunction, anticholinergic effects, anorexia, photosensitivity; neuroleptic malignant syndrome; cardiotoxicity; hepatotoxicity; agranulocytosis

(Continued text on following page)

Antimanic and Mood-Stabilizing Agents: Extreme Shifts in Emotions Between Mania and Depression

Mechanism of Action	Examples	Nontherapeutic Effects
Lithium: Affects neurotransmitters dopamine, serotonin, norepinephrine, acetylcholine, and GABA	lithium carbonate	Headache, fatigue, recent memory loss, anorexia, N&V, diarrhea, muscle weakness, dizziness ↓BP Toxic effect: slurred speech, ataxia, tremors, disorientation, confusion, severe thirst, cogwheel rigidity, dilute urine, tinnitus, respiratory depression, coma Teratogenic effect during first trimester
CNS agents, anti-seizure agents: Action varies depending on med	carbamazepine (Tegretol) gabapentin (Neurontin) lamotrigine (Lamictal) topiramate (Topamax) valproate (Depakote)	Drowsiness, fatigue, headache, nausea, blurred vision, psychomotor slowing; may cause ↓WBCs and ↑platelets

Nursing Implications

- Teach effect may take 1-2wk; sedation may occur immediately; avoid hazardous activities
- Obtain BP before each dose; hold drug based on systolic/diastolic parameters
- Limit exposure to sun; wear protective clothing, sunblock, sunglasses
- ↑Anticholinergic effects: ↑Fluids, fiber diet, hard candy
- Avoid coffee, tea, cola, antacids that ↓med effectiveness
- Monitor CBC and liver function studies routinely
- Monitor weight to assess response to anorexia and energy expenditure of EPS
- Assess for S&S of cardiotoxicity, particularly during initiation of therapy
- Assess for EPS; notify MD—effects may be reversible if dose is ↑ or withdrawn; some may be permanent
- Administer other med to ↓EPS: Benztropine (Cogentin), clonazepam (Klonopin), diazepam (Valium)
- Administer other meds to ↑neuroleptic malignant syndrome: amantadine (Symmetrel), bromocriptine (Parlodel)

Nursing Implications

- **Lithium**
  - Teach effect may take 1-2wk
  - Administer with meals to ↓GI irritation; do not crush/chew
  - Maintain fluid and Na intake; dehydration & hyponatremia lead to toxicity
  - Assess therapeutic blood levels (0.15-1.5mEq/L) wkly and then q2-3mo; has narrow therapeutic window
- **CNS and antiseizure agents:**
  - Ensure tabs are swallowed whole, chewable tabs chewed, sustained-release tabs not chewed/crushed, and carbonated beverages not used to dilute elixir
  - Avoid hazardous activities; protect from injury
  - Monitor CBC and platelet counts routinely

Medications for Attention Deficit Hyperactivity: ↓Hyperactivity, ↑Alertness, ↑Focus, ↓Distractibility

Mechanism of Action	Examples	Nontherapeutic Effects
CNS stimulants: Stimulate areas of the CNS, mainly cerebral cortex	methylphenidate (Concerta, Ritalin)	Anorexia, insomnia, hyper-sensitivity, tachycardia, palpitations, HTN, rest-lessness, wt loss, growth suppression; may cause paradoxical hyperactivity
Nonstimulant: Norepine-phrine reuptake inhibitor	atomoxetine (Strattera)	Headache, insomnia, anorexia, vomiting, abdominal pain, cough, irritability, aggression, impotence

Nursing Implications

- Give 30-45min ac to ↑food intake before anorexia occurs
- Give 6hr before hs to ↓sleep disturbances
- Obtain baseline and periodic wt for signs of ↓growth; dose determined by child's wt
- Assess for S&S of depression or aggression; may require D/C of med
- Inform school nurse and teacher of med regimen
- Teach that a drug holiday may be ordered to assess progress and ↓dependence
- Withdraw gradually with medical supervision

(Continued text on following page)

MEDS

- **CNS stimulants**
  - Teach duration is 3-6hr, 8hr for sustained-release forms
  - Avoid chewing/crushing of sustained-release tablets
- **Strattera**
  - Teach duration is 12-24hr

Nontherapeutic Effects of Psychotropic Meds

Agranulocytosis

- S & S of infection, fever, sore throat/cough
- Urinary frequency/urgency

Anticholinergic effects

- Dry mouth, urinary retention, constipation
- Blurred vision, ↑P

Cardiac toxicity

- S & S of heart failure↑, ↓BP, dysrhythmias, SOB, fatigue, ↓ weight
- Edema

CNS depression

- Drowsiness, sedation, orthostatic hypotension

Peripheral CNS stimulation (sympathomimetic)

- ↑P, ↑BP, tremor, dysrhythmias
- Restlessness, nightmares, insomnia, confusion

Extrapyramidal side effects (EPS)

- **Akathisia:** Motor agitation, inability to rest/relax, pacing, restless legs, compulsive movements
- **Dystonia:** Severe muscle spasms of back, neck, face, tongue
- **Parkinsonism:** Tremor, muscle rigidity, bradykinesia, masklike face, stooped posture, shuffling gait, drooling, restlessness
- **Tardive dyskinesia:** Involuntary movements of tongue and face (rolling or protrusion of tongue, lip smacking, teeth grinding, chewing motions, tics; movements disappear during sleep)

Hepatotoxicity

- Altered liver function studies; jaundice

Hypersensitivity

- Rash, fever, arthralgia, urticaria

Hypertensive crisis

- Caused by high dose antipsychotic meds or interactions
    - Headache, palpitations, stiff neck, photophobia, nausea
    - Flushing, diaphoresis, dysrhythmias, death

Hyponatremia

- N&V, diarrhea
- Fasciculations, stupor, seizures

Neuroleptic malignant syndrome

- Caused by dopamine blockade in hypothalamus due to ↑dose of antipsychotic meds
- Fever (cardinal sign), diaphoresis
- Muscle rigidity, drowsiness
- Unstable BP, ↓ventilation, dysrhythmias

Serotonin syndrome (SES)

- Caused by high dose of antidepressants; can be fatal
- Confusion, anxiety
- Hyperpyrexia, ataxia, restlessness, tremors
- Hypertension, sweating
- **Sexual dysfunction**
    - ↓Libido, ↓ability to reach orgasm, delayed ejaculation, impotence
    - Cessation of menses or ovulation

Antiseizure Agents: ↓Occurrence, Frequency, and/or Severity of Seizures

Seizure Type	Examples	Nontherapeutic Effects
Tonic-clonic	carbamazepine (Tegretol) gabapentin (Neurontin) phenytoin (Dilantin) phenobarbital (Luminal) valproic acid (Depakote)	Drowsiness, dizziness, N&V, rash, headache, ↓BP, respiratory depression, blood dyscrasias (↓WBC, ↓RBC, ↓platelets), hepatotoxicity
Absence	acetazolamide (Diamox)	**Phenytoin:** Ataxia, gingival hyperplasia, hirsutism, urine that is pink, red, or brown
Focal	lamotrigine (Lamictal) levetiracetam (Keppra) topiramate (Topamax)	

Nursing Implications

- Increase gradually as ordered until seizure control is achieved; control may require 2 antiseizure meds
- Shake suspensions before administration; give with food to ↓GI irritation
- Assess seizure activity: Precipitating event, presence of aura, specific origin and progression of motor activity, length, pt response

(Continued text on following page)

- Advise MD consult when planning pregnancy or lactation; some ↓effectiveness of oral contraceptives
- Provide oral hygiene
- Avoid hazardous activity; provide for safety during and after seizure
- Avoid alcohol and other CNS depressants
- Administer IV diazepam (Valium) or lorazepam (Ativan) as ordered for a prolonged/sustained tonic-clonic seizure (status epilepticus) keep resuscitative equipment available
- Monitor serum drug levels; phenytoin: therapeutic 10-20mcg/L, toxic 30-50mcg/L
- Seizures occur with abrupt withdrawal; withdraw med over 6-12wk
- Teach that med may be continued indefinitely; withdrawal may be attempted after 3yr of being seizure-free

Bone Resorption Inhibitors: ↓Bone Resorption, ↑Bone Density, ↓Potential for Fractures		
Drug Type and Mechanism of Action	**Examples**	**Nontherapeutic Effects**
Bisphosphonates: ↓Osteoclast activity, ↓bone resorption	alendronate (Fosamax) risedronate (Actonel) zoledronic acid (Zometa)	N&V, diarrhea, bone pain, abd pain, flushing; may cause osteonecrosis of jaw
Hormonal agents: Opposes effects of parathyroid hormone	calcitonin-salmon origin (Miacalcin)	Transient N&V, diarrhea, nasal irritation, flushing

Nursing Implications

- Teach effect takes >1mo
- Assess for hypocalcemia (↓BP, muscle spasms, paresthesias, laryngospasm, positive Chvostek or Trousseau signs)
- Discuss plans for pregnancy or lactation with MD
- Encourage intake of calcium foods, calcium and vitamin D supplements
- Encourage wt-bearing exercise; avoid smoking, alcohol, and cola, which ↑osteoporosis, ensure baseline bone density test
- **Calcitonin-salmon origin:** Perform intradermal allergy test first (drug may cause anaphylaxis); alternate nostrils daily with intranasal calcitonin; causes flushing/warmth for 1 hr after IM or sub-Q injection
- **Bisphosphonates:** Teach to take po dose in a.m. with water on empty stomach

Degenerative Diseases of the Nervous System

Parkinson's Disease: Restore Dopamine and Acetylcholine Balance; ↓Motor S&S (Stooped Posture, Nonintention Tremors, Rigidity, ↓Coordination)

Mechanism of Action	Examples	Nontherapeutic Effects
Dopaminergics: ↑Dopamine in corpus striatum	amantadine (Symmetrel) bromocriptine (Parlodel) carbidopa-levodopa (Sinemet)	↓BP, ↑P, fatigue, anorexia, N&V, dry mouth, constipation, tremors **Toxicity:** Muscle twitching, mood changes **Sinemet:** Urine and perspiration may darken in color
Anticholinergics: ↓Excess cholinergic activity in brain	benztropine (Cogentin)	Dry mouth, blurred vision, ↑pulse, constipation, urinary retention

Nursing Implications
- Do not D/C abruptly—Parkinsonian crisis may occur
- Teach effect may take several months; therapy is palliative
- Give exactly as ordered and slowly because of dysphagia
- Encourage eating after administration to take advantage of ↓in dysphagia and to ↓GI irritation
- Monitor VS; change position slowly; avoid hazardous activity
- **Dopaminergics:** ↓Effect with ↑pyridoxine (B₆) foods (veal, lamb, pork, egg yolks, potatoes). **Sinemet:** Avoid with narrow-angle glaucoma and MAO inhibitors
- **Anticholinergics:** Provide frequent oral care; encourage use of gum or hard candy to ↑salivation; stool softeners; catheterization may be necessary for retention

Alzheimer's Disease: ↓Progressive S&S of Dementia Related to Cognition, Behavior, ADL

Mechanism of Action	Examples	Nontherapeutic Effects
Acetylcholinesterase (AchE) inhibitors: ↑Acetylcholine levels in cerebral cortex	donepezil (Aricept) galantamine (Reminyl)	Anorexia, N&V, diarrhea, ↓BP, headache, dizziness, insomnia **Overdose:** Severe N&V, diaphoresis, salivation, ↓P, seizures, ↑muscle weakness (including respiratory muscles)

(Continued text on following page)

MEDS

Nursing Implications

- Use meds with caution in pts with COPD or asthma
- Teach therapy is palliative, not a cure; usually for rest of life
- Give with food/milk to ↓GI irritation; monitor wt wkly
- Monitor Hgb, Hct, and stool for melena
- Monitor VS, particularly BP, P, and respiratory status
- Protect from injury

Myasthenia Gravis: ↑Strength of Skeletal Muscle Contraction

Mechanism of Action	Examples	Nontherapeutic Effects
Anticholinesterase muscle stimulants: ↓Cholinesterase thus ↑acetylcholine	edrophonium (Tensilon) pyridostigmine (Mestinon)	Cholinergic S&S: lacrimation, salivation, N&V, diarrhea, intestinal cramping, ↓P, papillary constriction

Nursing Implications

- Monitor for dyspnea, dysphagia, dysarthria, and respiratory arrest (**myasthenic crisis**) or overdose of anticholinergic drugs (**cholinergic crisis**); give edrophonium as ordered to distinguish myasthenic crisis (S&S will ↓) from cholinergic crisis (S&S will ↑); keep IV atropine sulfate available as antidote for anticholinesterase muscle stimulants
- Administer carefully due to dysphagia
- Give meds exactly as scheduled; usually before meals to improve chewing/swallowing
- Give with food/milk to ↓GI irritation
- Monitor response as dosage is adjusted accordingly
- Balance activity/rest; plan activities when strength is greatest
- Have tracheostomy set and resuscitative equipment available

Cardiac Medications
Antidysrhythmics: ↓Abnormal Electrical Conduction Through Heart

Mechanism of Action	Examples	Nontherapeutic Effects
Class I—calcium ion antagonists: Slows conduction; local anesthetic; used for ventricular dysrhythmias	procainamide (Procanbid) lidocaine (Xylocaine)	Heart failure, new dysrhythmias, ↓BP, GI distress, blood dyscrasias, anticholinergic effects, diarrhea, neurotoxicity

Antidysrhythmics: ↓Abnormal Electrical Conduction Through Heart *(cont'd)*

Mechanism of Action	Examples	Nontherapeutic Effects
Class II—β-adrenergic blocker: ↓Cardiac excitability, output, and workload; ↓heart rate and ↓BP	metoprolol (Lopressor) propranolol (Inderal)	Heart failure, new dysrhythmias, ↓BP, GI distress, blood dyscrasias, anticholinergic effects, diarrhea, neurotoxicity
Class III—potassium channel blockers: Slows heart rate and conduction; used for ventricular and supraventricular dysrhthmias	amiodarone (Cordarone)	
Class IV—calcium channel blocker: ↓Entry of calcium into myocardial and vascular smooth muscle cells; ↓SA and AV node conduction; used for atrial fibrillation and supraventricular tachycardia	verapamil (Calan) diltiazem (Cardizem)	

Nursing Implications

- Keep resuscitative equipment available
- Use infusion controller when giving IV; monitor VS, BP, and ECG continually until stable
- Monitor HR before administration; withhold drug based on individually preset parameters
- Monitor therapeutic blood levels
- Monitor for ↑fluid volume (breath sounds, edema, wt gain)
- Maintain safety; change position slowly (↓hypotension)
- Teach about drug regimen, need to ↓Na intake, report side effects, identify irregular beats or ↑↓heart rate, need for continued medical supervision

Cardiac Glycosides: ↑Force of Cardiac Contraction, ↓Heart Rate, ↑Cardiac Output

Mechanism of Action	Example	Nontherapeutic Effects
Cardiac glycoside: Inhibits Na, K-adenosine triphosphatase → ↑ cardiac intracellular calcium and ↑ myocardial contractility	digoxin (Lanoxin)	↓P, headache, drowsiness, fatigue, weakness **Toxicity:** N&V, anorexia, visual disturbances (blurred, yellow vision), premature ventricular complexes, diarrhea

Nursing Implications
- Assess S&S of toxicity: ↓K⁺, ↑age → ↑ risk of toxicity
- Give loading dose initially (**digitalization**)
- Assess apical pulse; hold drug and notify MD if less than preset parameters (e.g., 50-60bpm)
- Monitor blood for therapeutic drug levels (0.8 to 2.0ng/mL)
- Monitor potassium (K⁺) levels; notify MD of hypokalemia below 3.5mEq/L
- Monitor for hyperkalemia if on potassium-sparing diuretic or corticosteroids
- Encourage foods ↑ in K⁺ unless taking K⁺ sparing med
- Teach to take pulse, recognize S&S of toxicity, and to call MD if S&S occur

Cardiac Stimulants: ↑Heart Rate

Mechanism of Action	Example	Nontherapeutic Effects
Cardiac stimulants: Stimulate alpha and beta receptors in the heart to ↑heart rate and contractility	atropine sulfate dobutamine (Dobutrex) norepinephrine (Levophed) epinephrine (Adrenalin)	Dysrhythmias, ↑P, headache, angina, anticholinergic effects

Nursing Implications
- Monitor VS, BP, frequently during administration
- Continuous ECG when giving IV
- Ensure ongoing follow-up care and ECGs

Coronary Vasodilators: Dilate Arteries, ↓Preload and Afterload, ↓Myocardial O₂ Consumption

Mechanism of Action	Example	Nontherapeutic Effects
Coronary vasodilators: Mechanism varies by drug; blocks calcium channels or relaxes smooth muscle to treat angina, mild hypertension	amlodipine (Norvasc) isosorbide mononitrate (Imdur) nifedipine (Procardia) nitroglycerine (Transderm-Nitro, Sublingual Nitrostat) verapamil (Calan)	Orthostatic hypotension, ↑P, headache, dizziness, N&V, flushing, confusion

Nursing Implications
- Assess BP; hold at individually set parameters
- **Nitroglycerine:** Teach to take sip of water, put sublingual tablet under tongue (may feel light tingling), take 1 pill every 5min up to 3 times for chest pain. If pain continues, get emergency help; store tablets in dark, tightly closed bottle; meds expire in 6mo; take acetaminophen for headache

Drug-Herb Interactions

Herb/Use	Interactions
Echinacea: Anti-infective, antipyretic	↑Hepatotoxicity with amiodarone, anabolic steroids, ketoconazole and methotrexate
Feverfew: Migraine headache	↑Bleeding potential with aspirin, heparin, NSAIDs and warfarin
Garlic: Lipid-lowering agent	↑Bleeding potential with aspirin, NSAIDs, and warfarin; ↑hypoglycemic effect of insulin and oral hypoglycemics
Ginger: Antiemetic	↑Bleeding potential with aspirin, heparin, NSAIDs and warfarin
Ginkgo: Antiplatelet agent, CNS stimulant	↑Bleeding potential with aspirin, heparin, NSAIDs and warfarin; ↓effect of anticonvulsants, tricyclic antidepressants
Ginseng: ↑Stamina, ↑immune response, ↑appetite; antidepressant	↓Anticoagulant effect of warfarin; ↑hypoglycemic effect of insulin and oral hypoglycemics; ↑digoxin toxicity; ↓effect of diuretics; ↑effect of CNS depressants

(Continued text on following page)

Herb/Use	Interactions
Kava kava: Antianxiety agent, sedative, hypnotic	↓Sedation with barbiturates, and benzodiazepines; CNS depressants, ↑dystonia with pheno-thiazines
St. John's wort: Antide-pressant	May cause serotonin syndrome with TCAs and SSRIs; may cause hypertensive crisis with MAO inhibitors; ↑sedation with CNS depressants: ↓effect of cyclosporine, reserpine, and theophylline; ↑anticoagulant effect of warfarin; ↓antiretroviral effect of protease inhibitors
Valerian: Antianxiety agent, sedative, hypnotic	↓Sedation with barbiturates, benzodiazepines, and CNS depressants

Medication Administration

Medication Administration—Key Points

5 Rights of Med Administration

✓ Right **patient** (check armband; follow agency policy)
✓ Right **medication**
✓ Right **dose**
✓ Right **route**
✓ Right **time**
✓ 6th Right: Is the drug still appropriate?

Patient Rights

✓ Right to refuse medication
✓ Right to be educated
✓ Right to administration by knowledgeable, licensed person
✓ Right not to receive experimental therapy without consent

Triple Check Before You Administer

■ **First:** Check label when removing from storage
■ **Second:** Compare med label to MAR
■ **Third:** Check again after med preparation, before administration

Patient Teaching

■ Assess pt attitude, self-administration skills
■ Provide clear oral and written instructions, use understandable language
■ Include family members
■ Evaluate learning, return demonstration

- Significant information to teach patient:
  - Generic and trade name, purpose, therapeutic effect
  - Dose, route, frequency, and when to take prn meds
  - Nontherapeutic effects and what to do if S&S occur
  - What to do if a dose is missed
  - Specific implications on how to store, to take with/without food, pre- and post-administration assessments

Safe Medication Administration

Preadministration Activities

- Check patient armband, MAR, and pt record for allergies
- Obtain history of prescription and OTC meds used
- Be informed: Check sources when unfamiliar with med
- Confirm written order; repeat back and have a witness for verbal or phone orders
- Question overdose or subtherapeutic dose
- Question med duplication or extended use
- Question med order without indication for use

Administration Activities

- Verify order against MAR
- Investigate compatibilities and interactions
- Calculate med dosage accurately; have another practitioner double check calculations
- Follow patient, administration rights, and triple check procedures
- Do not rush patient, ensure patient has ingested po medications
- Record meds administered
- Document reasons for nonadministered meds
- Evaluate patient's response (therapeutic, nontherapeutic)
- Notify MD of concerns or if patient vomits within 10min after ingestion

Safety and Legal Issues

- Do not borrow meds from another pt
- Give only meds personally prepared
- Do not leave meds at bedside
- Double lock controlled meds; have waste witnessed
- Use filtered needle when drawing meds from ampule
- Crush meds to facilitate ingestion; do not crush enteric or time-release meds; mix with smallest volume (applesauce)
- Never document before med is administered
- Document and report all med errors

Factors Affecting Med Therapy

Development
- **Infants:** Immaturity of liver and kidney require ↑dose
- **Older adults:** ↓Liver and kidney function → accumulation; ↓circulation and gastric function ← ↓med absorption; many meds (**polypharmacy**) ↑interactions
- **Pregnancy:** Some meds may cause abnormal development of embryo (**teratogenic effect**)
- **Diet:** Nutrients can ↑or↓ absorption or action of med
- **Gender:** Distribution of body fat/fluid/hormones affect med action
- **Environment:** Environmental temperature can ↑or ↓peripheral vasoconstriction altering med action; noise can interfere with effect of sedatives/analgesics
- **Pathology:** ↓Liver or kidney function cause ↑med accumulation; ↓gastric or ↓circulatory function cause ↑med absorption
- **Time of administration:** ↑Absorption on empty stomach; with food ↓to ↓GI distress; circadian and sleep cycles can affect response
- **Body weight:** Dose calculated by pt's wt or body surface area
- **Genetic/ethnic:** Usual dose may be toxic; herbal treatments may interfere with med therapy; Asians may need ↓dose of antipsychotic and antianxiety meds [2] slower metabolism of these drugs; African Americans may need ↑dose of antihypertensives
- **Psychological issues:** pt's positive/negative expectations can ↑↓response

Effects of Meds

- **Adverse effect:** Severe side effect or toxicity
- **Allergic reaction:** Immunological reaction
- **Anaphylactic reaction:** Hypersensitive, life-threatening reaction
- **Cumulative effect:** Excessive level of med in body when intake is higher than metabolism or excretion
- **Drug abuse:** Inappropriate intake of a med
- **Drug dependence:** Psychological/physiological need to take a med
- **Drug habituation:** Mild form of psychological dependence
- **Drug interaction:** When 1 med alters the effect of 1 or more meds
- **Drug tolerance:** Requiring ↑dose to achieve therapeutic effect
- **Drug toxicity:** Dangerous effect [2] excessive dose
- **Idiosyncratic effect:** Unexpected or unique response
- **Inhibiting effect:** 1 med decreases effect of another med
- **Potentiating/synergistic effect:** 1 med adds to, prolongs, or ↑action of another med
- **Side effect:** Predictable nontherapeutic effect that is tolerable
- **Therapeutic/desired effect:** Reason med was prescribed

Medication Administration Routes

Route	Advantages (Pro) and Disadvantages (Con)	Nursing Care
Buccal Tablet held between cheek and gum until dissolved; local effect Absorbed within mins	**Pro:** Rapid relief **Con:** Remains until dissolved; can be swallowed, chewed, or aspirated accidentally	Alternate cheeks to avoid mucosal irritation Warn not to chew/swallow tablet or sleep until dissolved to ↓risk of aspiration
Nasogastric tube (NGT), gastrostomy tube (GT, PEG) Instillation of med via a tube into stomach	**Pro:** Used for ↓gag reflex and unconscious pts **Con:** Risk for aspiration Requires intact enteral tube and special equipment	↑HOB, ensure placement of tube in stomach (aspirate gastric contents), clear tube with 30mL of water, insert med through tube, clear tube with 30mL of water after Assess for aspiration
Inhalation Meds dispersed through aerosolized solution or powder that penetrates airways rapidly promoting absorption **MDI:** Metered-dose inhaler (MDI) **NPA:** Nonpressurized aerosol (nebulizer) **DPI:** Dry powdered inhaler	**Pro:** Rapid effect; can be given to unconscious pt **Con:** Can cause undesired systemic effects Equipment needs to be cleaned and stored Pt with ↓cognition, infants, or children may be unable to follow directions MDI requires coordination with inhalation and device compression	**MDI:** Shake canister before each depression; exhale through pursed lips; hold 2cm from mouth or insert mouthpiece beyond teeth with lips around mouthpiece; depress device while inhaling slowly/deeply; hold breath 5-10sec; exhale slowly via pursed lips; wait 1-2min between inhalations; use of spacer (extender) ↓particle size → ↑absorption and ↓droplets on tongue; rinse mouth after administration of steroids **DPI:** Dose in chamber is aerosolized when inhaled **NPA:** Insert dose in chamber; breathe in and out with lips closed around mouthpiece; repeat until no mist is seen; take 1 deep breath q5breaths

(Continued text on following page)

Route	Advantages (Pro) and Disadvantages (Con)	Nursing Care
Intradermal (ID) Solution injected into dermis just under epidermis Slow absorption Volume 0.1-0.3mL	**Pro:** Used for allergy testing **Con:** Pierces skin	Use standard precautions; assess for allergic/ anaphylactic reaction when used for allergy testing
Intramuscular (IM) Solution injected into muscle Onset 3-5min Volume 1-3mL	**Pro:** Used when oral route is contraindicated; more rapidly absorbed than oral, topical, or sub-Q **Con:** Pierces skin; more tissue damage than Sub-Q Requires adequate peripheral circulation Can cause anxiety	Use standard precautions Use sterile technique Position pt to access injection site Rotate sites; landmark sites
Intravenous (IV) Solution injected into intravascular compartment via a vein Immediate onset	**Pro:** Immediate therapeutic effect **Con:** ↑Cost than oral Can cause anxiety	Use standard precautions Use sterile technique IV push, intermittent, continuous titrated drips Change tubing every 24-72hr and site 3-7 days as per agency policy
Oral (PO) Taken by mouth (tablet, capsule, liquid) Absorbed in GI tract Onset 30-45min	**Pro:** Convenient, does not invade skin, economical; less psychological stress than other routes **Con:** May irritate gastric mucosa, have bad taste/odor, discolor or erode teeth, cause aspiration **Contraindications:** Vomiting, dysphasia, unconsciousness, before special testing, continuous NG suction	↓HOB to ensure safe swallowing Pace intake to ↓aspiration if difficulty swallowing; crush and mix with food (contraindicated for extended release and enteric coated meds) or obtain liquid form if available Obtain order for alternate route

Medication Administration Routes *(Continued)*		
Route	**Advantages (Pro) and Disadvantages (Con)**	**Nursing Care**
Rectal (PR) Suppository or solution inserted into anus Slow absorption; local or systemic effect	**Pro:** Local effect Used if oral route is contraindicated **Con:** Embarrassing Absorption unpredictable **Contraindications:** In rectal surgery or rectal bleeding	Use standard precautions Position pt in lateral or Sim's position for insertion
Subcutaneous (Sub-Q) Tissue just below skin Onset 3-20min Volume ≤ 1mL	**Pro:** Faster than oral **Con:** Pierces skin Can be irritating to tissue	Use standard precautions Use sterile technique Rotate injection sites Landmark sites
Sublingual (SL) Under tongue Rapid absorption	**Pro:** Immediate therapeutic response **Con:** Can be swallowed, chewed, or aspirated accidentally	Instruct pt to keep liquid/tablet under tongue Warn not to chew/swallow tablet or sleep until it is absorbed
Buccal Solid med placed against mucous membranes of cheek Slow absorption Local or systemic effect	**Pro:** Slowly dissolved med is swallowed with saliva **Con:** Can be swallowed, chewed, or aspirated accidentally	Instruct pt to keep tablet (troche, lozenge) against mucous membranes of cheek and alternate cheeks Warn not to chew/swallow tablet or sleep until it is absorbed
Transdermal (Percutaneous) Via skin Prolonged systemic effect	**Pro:** Limited side effects; avoids GI irritation **Con:** Residue may soil clothes or irritate skin	Wear gloves to ↓self-contamination Use site indicated by manufacturer (chest, upper arms, anterior thighs); rotate sites Avoid impaired skin; use hairless area to ↑patch contact) Wash site after removing patch

(Continued text on following page)

Route	Advantages (Pro) and Disadvantages (Con)	Nursing Care
Vaginal Inserted into vaginal vault	**Pro:** Local effect **Con:** Limited use, embarrassment	Use standard precautions Provide perineal care before and after Position in dorsal recumbent or Sim's position Insert applicator 2inches into vagina and depress plunger Instruct to remain supine for 15min Wash applicator

Intramuscular Injection Sites and Z-Track Method for Giving IM Injections

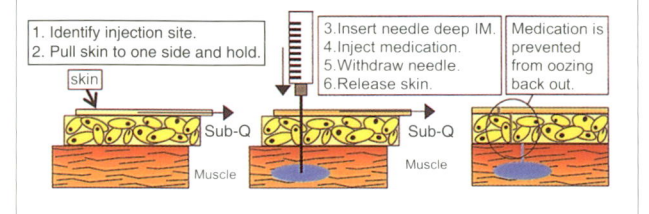

1. Identify injection site.
2. Pull skin to one side and hold.

skin

Sub-Q

Muscle

3. Insert needle deep IM.
4. Inject medication.
5. Withdraw needle.
6. Release skin.

Sub-Q

Muscle

Medication is prevented from oozing back out.

Intradermal (ID), Subcutaneous (Sub-Q), and Intramuscular (IM)

	ID	Sub-Q	IM
Site	Inner forearm, chest, and back	Outer upper arm, anterior thigh, and abdomen	Gluteus, thigh, and deltoid muscles
Gauge and Length	27–30 g 1/4–3/8"	25–28 g 5/8"	23 g 1–1½"
Angle	10–15°	90° 45° for very thin patients	90°
Volume	0.1–0.2 mL	0.5–1 mL	Up to 3 mL; small muscles (deltoid) no more than 1 mL

Sub-Q Heparin Injections

Site	Gauge and Angle	Aspirate	Message Site
Abdomen, posterior upper arm, low back, thigh, and upper back	25 g–26 g. 3/8" @ 90° (45° if on a thin patient)	No	No

Subcutaneous (Sub-Q) Injection Sites and IM and Sub-Q Injection Techniques

Subcutaneous Injection Sites	IM and Sub-Q Techniques
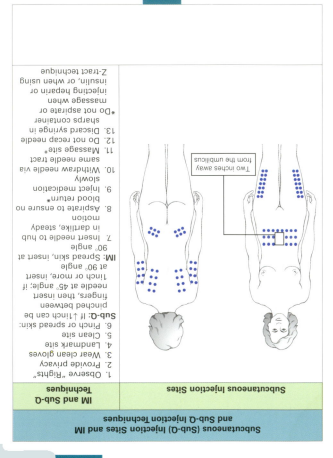	1. Observe "Rights" 2. Provide privacy 3. Wear clean gloves 4. Landmark site 5. Clean site 6. Pinch or spread skin: **Sub-Q:** If ↑ 1 inch can be pinched between fingers, then insert needle at 45° angle; if 1 inch or more, insert at 90° angle **IM:** Spread skin, insert at 90° angle 7. Insert needle to hub in dartlike, steady motion 8. Aspirate to ensure no blood return* 9. Inject medication slowly 10. Withdraw needle via same needle tract 11. Massage site* 12. Do not recap needle 13. Discard syringe in sharps container *Do not aspirate or massage when injecting heparin or insulin, or when using Z-tract technique

Two inches away from the umbilicus

IV Piggyback (IVPB) Setup

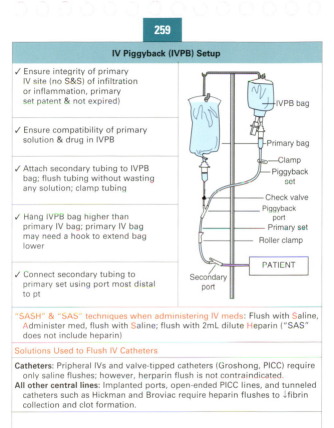

✓ Ensure integrity of primary IV site (no S&S) of infiltration or inflammation, primary set patent & not expired)

✓ Ensure compatibility of primary solution & drug in IVPB

✓ Attach secondary tubing to IVPB bag; flush tubing without wasting any solution; clamp tubing

✓ Hang IVPB bag higher than primary IV bag; primary IV bag may need a hook to extend bag lower

✓ Connect secondary tubing to primary set using port most distal to pt

Labels on diagram: IVPB bag, Primary bag, Clamp, Piggyback set, Check valve, Piggyback port, Primary set, Roller clamp, PATIENT, Secondary port

"SASH" & "SAS" techniques when administering IV meds: Flush with Saline, Administer med, flush with Saline; flush with 2mL dilute Heparin ("SAS" does not include heparin)

Solutions Used to Flush IV Catheters

Catheters: Pripheral IVs and valve-tipped catheters (Groshong, PICC) require only saline flushes; however, herparin flush is not contraindicated.
All other central lines: Implanted ports, open-ended PICC lines, and tunneled catheters such as Hickman and Broviac require heparin flushes to ↓fibrin collection and clot formation.

Complications of IV Therapy

Complication	Assessment	Nursing Interventions
Infiltration: IV fluid escapes into subcutaneous tissue; ↓ or no fluids infusing	Assess site for swelling, pale, cool to touch. No blood backflash	D/C IV and apply warm compress (needs order) Restart in new site **Prevention:** Discourage movement of limb with IV
Phlebitis: Inflammation of vein **Thrombus:** Blood clot; IV flow may stop due to obstruction	Assess for red line/burning pain along course of vein, heat, and swelling	D/C IV, apply warm compress (need order), do not massage or rub affected area; notify MD Restart in new site **Prevention:** Discourage movement of limb with IV flush as per policy, rotate sites every 72-96hr
Fluid overload: Rate is faster than ordered; patient cannot tolerate rate of infusion	Assess for hypervole-mia: bounding, P; ↓BP, ↑R, lung base crackles, dyspnea, distended neck veins	↓IV rate; notify MD If experiencing respiratory complications, ↑HOB and provide O₂ at 2L **Prevention:** Monitor rate regularly; use time tape and volume control device
Incorrect IV solution is infusing	Check MD IV order against hanging IV fluid	↓IV rate to maintain patency; immediately hang correct solution; notify MD Record and complete incident report **Prevention:** Verify IV solution against MD order 3 times before hanging IV solution
IV rate is too slow: Volume absorbed is less than ordered	Inspect factors affecting flow: kinks, lying on tubing, bag too low, arm position that ↑flow rate	Set at ordered rate, ensure bag is 3ft above IV site, coil tubing on bed surface, remove tubing from under pt, reposition arm **Prevention:** Monitor rate routinely, use time tape, discourage movement of limb with IV

Complications of IV Therapy *(Continued)*		
Complication	**Assessment**	**Nursing Interventions**
Air embolus: Air in intravascular compartment	Assess for respiratory distress, ↑P, cyanosis, ↓BP, ↓LOC	Secure system to prevent entry of air, place patient on left side in modified Trendelenburg position, monitor VS and pulse oximetry Notify MD immediately ***Prevention:*** Flush IV lines of air before use; secure and monitor integrity of system frequently
Sepsis: Systemic infection	Monitor for ↑VS and/or red, tender, insertion site	Follow agency guidelines for cultures (blood, exudate) Notify MD ***Prevention:*** Use meticulous sterile technique
Speed shock: response to fluids entering circulation too rapidly	Assess for ↑P, ↓BP, chills, flushed face, headache, chest tightness, dyspnea, back pain, ↓LOC, fainting Assess site for swelling, pale, cool to touch No blood backflash Assess for red line/burning pain along course of vein, heat, and swelling	D/C IV, notify MD, monitor VS ***Prevention:*** Monitor response first 15-30min frequently after hanging new solution/med, monitor rate frequently, use time tape and volume control pump

Medication Calculation Formulas

IV Drop Rate Formula

■ Drop factor equals number of drops per mL delivered by IV tubing

Drops per minute =
$$\frac{\text{(total volume in drops)}}{\text{(total time in minutes)}} \quad \frac{\text{total mL} \times \text{drop factor}}{1 \text{ hour} \times 60 \text{ minutes}}$$

Conversion of Pounds to Kilograms (Kg)

■ Solve for X by cross multiplying
■ Divide both sides of resulting equation by the number in front of the X
■ Reduce to lowest terms to achieve child's wt in kg

$$\frac{\text{child's weight in pounds}}{2.2 \text{ pounds}} = \frac{X \text{ kg}}{1 \text{ kg}}$$

Weight Based Method to Calculate a Pediatric Dose

$$\text{Pediatric dose in mg} = \frac{\text{Child's weight in kg}}{50 \text{ kg}} \times \text{Adult dose in mg}$$

Ratio and Proportion Formulas

- Ordered dose and dose on hand must be in same unit of measure
- **Formulas 1 and 2:** Solve for X by cross multiplying
- **Formula 3:** Solve for X by multiplying the means and the extremes
- Divide both sides of all resulting equations by the number in front of the X
- Reduce to lowest terms to achieve the quantity of dose

#1
$$\frac{desired}{have} = \frac{ordered\ dose}{dose\ on\ hand} = \frac{X\ quantity\ desired}{quantity\ on\ hand}$$

#2
$$\frac{quantity\ on\ hand}{dose\ on\ hand} = \frac{X\ quantity\ desired}{ordered\ dose}$$

#3
dose on hand : quantity on hand : : ordered dose : X quantity desired
(extreme)   (means)   (means)   (extremes)

Body Surface Area (BSA) Method to Calculate Pediatric Dose for Infants and Children ≤12 Years

- *Estimate the child's BSA in square meters (m^2) by using a BSA chart (nomogram).
- The **BSA chart** consists of three columns. The left column is height, the middle column is body surface area, and the right column is weight. These numbers ↑from the bottom to the top of each column.
- Draw a straight line from the child's height in the left column to the child's weight in the right column. The number found where the line crosses the middle column is the child's estimated BSA.
- The BSA should be used in the formula for the body surface area method to calculate a pediatric dose

Pediatric dose in mg = $\dfrac{\text{*Child's BSA in square meters } (m^2)}{1.73\ m^2} \times$ Adult dose in mg

Test Analysis Tools

Introduction

- This tab includes tips and analysis tools that will help you pass the NCLEX-RN®.
- Seven test-analysis tools will help you analyze the answers you get wrong on tests
- **Performance trends & information processing errors** focus on the *process* of test-taking and corrective action plans are presented to address your identified deficits
- **Knowledge deficits: universal information** focuses on content common to all disciplines in nursing practice
- Four tools concerning knowledge deficits **medical-surgical, pediatric, childbearing,** and **mental health/psychiatric nursing,** focus on discipline-specific content

Instructions

All tools except Performance Trends

- First look over each tool. After taking and scoring your test, use the tools to help you identify your area of weakness.
- Complete all tools in the same way:
  1. Place the number of a question you got wrong in a shaded box in the top row under **question number.**
  2. Identify the **processing error** or **knowledge category** associated with your error in the left column.
  3. Put a mark in the box where the row & column intersect on the chart; follow the first three steps for all your wrong answers.
  4. Tally the total number of marks for each row in the last column on the right; after you identify clusters of deficits, see the tool **corrective action plan** and follow the suggestions addressing your specific deficit.

Instructions for Performance Trends

- Answer the following questions to identify opportunities to improve your test-taking skills:

1. I am able to focus with little distraction	Yes ( ) No ( )
2. I feel calm and in control	Yes ( ) No ( )
3. I effectively use Test-Taking Techniques to reduce options	Yes ( ) No ( )
4. I change answers from wrong to right	Yes ( ) No ( )
5. I have no error clusters: 1st, middle, or end of exam	Yes ( ) No ( )

- If you answered No to any of these questions, see the tool **corrective action plan.**

Information Processing Score

Knowledge Category	Question Numbers								
Stem									
Missed negative polarity									
Missed word setting priority									
Missed important clues									
Misinterpreted information									
Missed central point, theme									
Read into the question									
Missed step in nursing process									
Incompletely analyzed stem									
Did not understand question									
Did not know the content									
Options									
Selected the answer too quickly									
Misidentified the priority									
Misinterpreted information									
Read into options									
Did not know the content									
Misapplied concepts, principles									
Transcribed incorrectly									

TOOLS

Knowledge Deficits: Universal Information

Knowledge Category	Question Numbers							
A&P and pathophysiology								
Basic care (including pain)								
Community care								
Complementary, alternative care								
Death/dying/loss/grief								
Emergency care								
Fluid and electrolyte balance								
Growth and development								
Inflammation/infection								
Leadership and management								
Legal and ethical issues								
Perioperative								
Pharmacology								
Psychosocial and communication								
Safety (physical/microbiologic)								
Teaching and learning								
Nursing Process								
Assessment								
Analysis and diagnosis								
Planning								
Implementation								
Evaluation								

Knowledge Category	Question Numbers								
Cardiac									
Endocrine									
Gastrointestinal, accessory organs of digestion (gallbladder, liver, pancreas)									
Gastrointestinal, upper (oral, esophageal, and gastric)									
Gastrointestinal, lower (small and large intestines)									
Hematologic, immunologic									
Integumentary									
Musculoskeletal									
Neoplastic									
Neurologic									
Peripheral vascular, lymphatic									
Reproductive (female)									
Reproductive (male)									
Respiratory									
Urinary tract, renal									
Other									

Knowledge Deficits: Pediatric Nursing									
Knowledge Category	**Question Numbers**								
Cardiac disease (congenital or acquired)									
Endocrine									
Gastrointestinal, accessory organs of digestion (gallbladder, liver, pancreas)									
Gastrointestinal, upper (oral, esophageal, gastric)									
Gastrointestinal, lower (small, large intestines)									
Genital/urinary/renal									
Growth and development									
Health promotion and immunization									
Hematological and immunological									
Integumentary									
Musculoskeletal									
Neoplastic									
Neurological									
Peripheral vascular and lymphatic									
Respiratory									
Other:									

Knowledge Category	Question Numbers
Family (adjustment/loss)	
Diagnostic testing	
Nutrition: maternal, infant (breast/formula)	
Prenatal care	
Intrapartal care (labor/birth)	
High-risk pregnancy	
Obstetric emergencies	
Postpartum care	
Healthy newborn	
High-risk newborn	
Other:	

Knowledge Category	Question Numbers
Crisis/stress management	
Defense mechanisms	
Dysfunctional behavior patterns	
Therapeutic communication	
Treatment modalities	
Violence (sexual/domestic/suicide)	
Other:	
Disorders	
Anxiety disorders	
Attention deficit and disruptive behavior	
Cognitive disorders (dementia/delirium)	
Dissociative disorders	

(Continued text on following page)

TOOLS

Knowledge Category	Question Numbers								
Eating disorders									
Factitious disorders									
Grief and loss									
Mood disorders (depressive/ bipolar)									
Personality disorders									
Pervasive developmental disorders									
Schizophrenia									
Sexual and gender identity disorders									
Somatoform disorders									
Substance abuse disorders									

Corrective Action Plan

Performance Trends

- Implement recommendations if you scored *No* on Performance Trends tool
  1. Be comfortable, rested, sit in area free of distractions; wear earplugs
  2. Develop a positive mental attitude (challenge negative thoughts, use positive self-talk: "I can do this!")
     - Regain control (use deep breathing, imagery, muscle relaxation)
     - Desensitize yourself to fear response (practice test-taking)
     - Establish control on day of exam (manage routine, travel, environment, supplies)
     - Stop exam, take a break, and regain control; belabor answering questions on content you do not know; overprepare for the exam
  3. Practice Test-Taking Tips presented in Tab 1
  4. If you change more answers from right to wrong on practice tests, *do not* change your first answer unless you are absolutely certain that the new answer is correct
  5. Use anxiety-reducing techniques during exam at times when error clusters appeared in practice; if due to fatigue, stop exam and take a short break; work at practice tests longer to ↑stamina

Information Processing Errors

■ Practice Test-Taking Tips presented in Tab 1
■ For more detail see: Nugent, *Test Success: Test-Taking Techniques for Beginning Nursing Students*, F.A. Davis Co., Philadelphia

Knowledge Deficits: All Areas

■ Focus study on clustered gaps in knowledge
■ Review notes, text, computer-assisted instruction, videos, practice test questions, and rationales, and use study books/workbooks
■ Do not waste time studying areas you know
■ Explore the F. A. Davis *Notes* series for a title that reviews the topic in more depth than is presented in NCLEX Notes (e.g., *Psych, MedSurg, Lab, MED, Ortho, Nutri, ECG, IV Therapy, RN*)

Notes

USER NAME: Krista 4711

PASSWORD: 6Dolphins